77

Ways to Beat
Colds and Flu

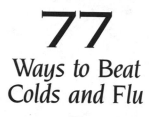

■

77

Ways to Beat Colds and Flu

■

Charles B. Inlander
and
Cynthia K. Moran

A *People's Medical Society* Book

WALKER AND COMPANY
NEW YORK

A note to the reader: The ideas, procedures, and suggestions contained in this book are not intended as a substitute for consulting with your practitioner. All matters regarding your health require medical supervision.

First published in the United States of America in 1994 by Walker Publishing Company, Inc.

Published simultaneously in Canada by Thomas Allen & Son Canada, Limited, Markham, Ontario

Library of Congress Cataloging-in-Publication Data

Inlander, Charles B.

77 ways to beat colds and flu / Charles B. Inlander and Cynthia K. Moran.

p. cm.

ISBN 0-8027-1304-1. — ISBN 0-8027-7447-4 (pbk.)

1. Cold (Disease)—Prevention. 2. Cold (Disease)—Treatment.

3. Cold (Disease)—Popular works. 4. Influenza—Prevention. 5. Influenza—Treatment.

6. Influenza—Popular works. I. Moran, Cynthia K. II. Title.

III. Title: Seventy-seven ways to beat colds and flu.

RF361.I55 1994

616.2'05—dc20

94-32102

CIP

Printed in the United States of America

2 4 6 8 10 9 7 5 3

■ CONTENTS

■ INTRODUCTION

When you think about how far medical science has progressed in the 20th century, it is hard to believe that colds and flu have not been eradicated. In the United States alone, more than $1 trillion a year is being spent on health care, yet the average American will suffer through at least two colds in those same 12 months. Millions will also endure one or more bouts of the flu.

As you will learn in 77 WAYS TO BEAT COLDS AND FLU, both are relatively complicated illnesses that have defied cure. Yet much is known about how to lower your chances of getting a cold or flu and even more is known about how to ease the misery that comes with them.

That is why the People's Medical Society has produced this book. As the nation's largest nonprofit consumer health advocacy organization, our major goal is to put information into your hands that will help you make the most informed health and medical decisions possible.

Based on the latest medical research, 77 WAYS TO BEAT COLDS AND FLU provides up-to-date information in simple, easy-to-read tips. So, while the medical researchers look for the cure, you can be taking charge in your own battle to prevent and ease the misery of two of the world's oldest ailments.

Charles B. Inlander, President
People's Medical Society

1 ■ Understanding Colds and Flu

They have been humanity's miserable enigma at least since written history began. In English-speaking countries we have come to call them the common cold and the flu.

Ancient civilizations knew colds as *katarrhein*, from the Greek, meaning "to flow down." In English *catarrh* refers to an inflammation of the mucous membrane in the nose and throat. But in the last century, "cold" was the moniker anointed in Great Britain because acquiring mucus-filled congestion–or "catching cold"–was blamed on England's cold, damp weather.

We adapted the term influenza, or the flu, from fourteenth-century Italy, when an unusual conjunction of planets was thought to "influenze" a rash of colds, fever, and coughs in earthbound humans. Several hundred years later, during the European epidemic of 1743, Latin writers penned influenza into the history books.

It wasn't until 1954 that researchers identified the actual viruses that cause colds and flu. We're still finding out about specific strains of these viruses. So far, we know of more than 200, from 20 different viral families. In 1994 the number we've identified is still growing, and our noses are still running.

We know that colds and flu come from viruses. We also know neither has a cure. If you're determined to combat them–or at least to reduce their miserable effects on you when they do strike–you'll need to have the answers to the following questions.

What's the difference between viruses and bacteria?

Viruses and bacteria rank among the world's smallest microscopic organisms. Bacteria, which do not cause colds or flu but can cause secondary problems, originated in the oceans millions of years ago. They are some of the simplest and oldest single-celled beings known to humanity. They exist throughout our environment, in oceans, lakes, and other moist settings. Some bacteria are beneficial, as are the molds in blue cheese and penicillin, while others are harmful – or pathogenic – causing disease to the human body. Bacteria reproduce rapidly by simple cell division, dividing in two, then in two again.

Viruses are much smaller. These submicroscopic organisms measure anywhere from 1/2 to 1/1000th the size of the smallest bacterium. None is beneficial. All viruses cause disease, including colds and flu. A virus is a parasite that can't reproduce on its own: It invades a host cell and commandeers the host's genetic material as its own by breaking down the host cell's molecular structure and merging with it. In its reproductive process, a virus destroys the host cell.

All viruses and bacteria reproduce prolifically. Under ideal conditions, a bacterium can divide every 20 minutes, which means that in 24 hours one bacterium can have 16 million offspring. Viruses self-replicate just as rapidly. Thus, when you are fighting a viral or bacterial infection, time is *not* on your side. Consequently, it's important to know what symptoms bacterial and viral invasions initiate so that you know how to treat your infections.

Unlike allergies, neither viruses nor bacteria are seasonal. Both can cause fever. A bacterial infection is differentiated from a virus by its single major symptom such as a phlegm-filled cough, an earache, or a sinus pain. In contrast, a virus usually has multiple symptoms that may include a runny nose, headache, muscle aches, dizziness, dry cough, and hoarseness. Antibiotics fight bacteria, but they do not work against viruses.

How do viruses and bacteria make me sick?

Bacteria produce poisons that are harmful to your cells. If they multiply rapidly enough, the poisons overwhelm your immune response, and you get sick. Viruses make you sick in one of several ways. Once you are invaded by a virus, your immune system may react symptomatically (prompting a cough or a sore throat) or with a disease process (producing antibodies that attach to the germs they're fighting as both travel throughout the body). Viruses can destroy or damage vital organs they invade. Or by changing (mutating) the genetic characters of some of your genes, viruses can cause cancer. Finally, a viral invasion can weaken your immune system to a point where you become more susceptible to other infections that your body cannot fight simultaneously.

Bacteria and viruses may enter the body the same way, through direct contact with some part of the respiratory system. Bacteria are more versatile than viruses, and can enter the body on food, through the urogenital tract or other skin openings, including open wounds. Once bacteria invade the body, they live on or near the skin where it's warm, moist, and near an oxygen source, all of which they need in order to multiply. Viruses also tend to stay close to where they enter the body. Some viruses, including those that cause colds and flu, produce symptoms quickly, while others—such as the virus that causes AIDS—may lie dormant for months or years before starting an infection.

Why are so many viral infections like colds and flu incurable?

A virus is a parasite that moves in with and becomes part of its host's cellular makeup. Scientists have had a difficult time discovering medical treatment that kills the virus without also killing the host cell. Some of the more successful antiviral medications, such as polio vaccine and amantadine, immobilize the virus they attack. Rather than killing it, this approach keeps a virus from reproducing.

With bacteria, on the other hand, it's possible to develop medications that attack the strain of bacteria directly and kill it. Other types of antibiotics prevent multiplication of the invader. When a vaccine or other medication successfully immobilizes a bacterium or virus, the action allows your immune system to overcome the invading germs and drive the pathogens from the body.

The huge number of viruses, each with the ability to mutate— or alter genetic structure—overwhelms and makes impractical the search for virus-specific cures. Although medical research is making great progress toward developing an antiviral drug that disables a whole class of viruses, until that happens, the most likely prospect for eradicating one from the body is through your own immune responses.

How does the flu differ from a cold?

Colds and the flu are caused by viruses. Multiple cold and flu viruses exist, which explains why some colds or cases of flu last longer or seem milder or have more symptoms than others. Of the 20 identified major virus families, most colds come from five. Three other viral families produce flu—identified as A, B, or C strains or types.

Type B and Type C flu are generally mild in adults: Both can be confused with bad colds. Once a person has a Type C flu, immunity accrues for life, so repeat attacks in the same person are rare. (Young children are especially susceptible to Type C flu, and their cases can be particularly serious.)

Type A flu is the least stable and the most volatile when it comes to mutating. Because it can alter its genetic makeup so frequently, immunity to Type A is neither significant nor long lasting. Thus, Type A flu strains—which cause more severe symptoms than a cold (a higher fever, extreme fatigue, and system-wide respiratory congestion)—are the flu viruses of epidemics and pandemics.

Most colds come from one of five virus families, although almost half come from the rhinovirus family. These viruses are so small that it wasn't until the late 1980s that scientists even got to see one.

A cold is known as an upper respiratory infection, which means it's restricted to the nose, throat, and surrounding air passages. Most colds are not accompanied by fever, chills, or the more severe symptoms identified with flu.

Flu, most notably a Type A strain, is almost always more severe than a cold. The defining characteristics that separate flu from a cold are its sudden arrival, usually heralded by a high fever and chills.

The two share the symptoms of fatigue, coughing, and nasal congestion. In a typical case, each bout of flu runs its course in almost the same length of time: just about a week (although residual weakness, lack of energy, and depression can last up to several weeks after most symptoms have passed). Generally, a person takes less time to rebound after a cold.

Virus Families Responsible for Most Colds

VIRUS FAMILY	% COLDS	SEASON(S)	IDENTIFYING FEATURES
Rhinovirus	40+	Spring through Fall	Nasal congestion in respiratory tract; no fever. lasts week or more; direct contact spreading; 120+ viruses in family.
Coronavirus	10-20	Coldest Months of Winter & Spring	Sneezing, runny nose; brief, over in 2 days, or can last 6-7; virus eludes immune system so can re-catch; fecal/oral spreading; pneumonia danger for children; significant outbreaks in 2-year intervals; aerosol spreading (sneezing, coughing); 13 known viruses in family.
Adenovirus	10	Cooler Months	Fever, sore throat with yellowish patches on tonsils (settles in adenoids, hence its name); pink eye; several strains cause gastroenteritis ("stomach flu"); 3 types cause 5% of all colds; fecal/oral spreading; viruses shed only 4 days; children highly susceptible; 40 known viruses in family.
Enterovirus	5-10	Spring through Fall (Peak: Summer & Fall)	Fever, sniffles, sore throat; diarrhea possible; some settle in digestive system; cold-causing subgroups: echoviruses (spread various ways), Coxsackie virus (aerosol spreading); also cause "summer colds"; dangerous complications include inflammation of heart, lung, brain; polio from this family; 7-14 day incubation period longest of all viral families; 125+ viruses in family.
Respiratory Syncytial Virus & Parainfluenza Virus	5-10 in adults	Fall through Spring	Mild in adults; lasts 5 days to week; immunity lasts a year; incubates in 3-6 days in adults, shedding stops after 8-10; aerosol, direct contact spreading; Virazole an effective drug against this family of viruses; 4 known viruses in family.

Is it a cold or the flu?

SYMPTOMS	COLD	FLU
Fever	Rare	Characteristics: high fever (102°-104°+); lasts 3-4 days
Headache	Rare	Prominent
General aches, pains	Slight	Usual; often severe
Fatigue; weakness	Quite mild	Can last up to 2-3 weeks
Prostration (extreme exhaustion)	Never	Early and prominent
Stuffy nose	Common	Sometimes
Sneezing	Usual	Sometimes
Sore throat	Common	Sometimes
Chest discomfort, cough	Mild to moderate; hacking cough	Common; can become severe

Source: National Institutes of Health

Is there a bad time of year for catching colds and flu? How long does each last? How long is a person contagious?

In the temperate zones, where most U.S. colds and flu are experienced, the peak of the cold and flu season occurs in the colder months, from November through February. Timing of the season is not a feature of cold weather itself, say scientists; rather it's the time when most of us remain indoors for longer stretches because of the weather.

Staying indoors exposes you to central heating systems, which are known for their drying effects on the mucous membranes, your first line of defense against viruses. Remaining in groups or crowds of people where contagious viral contact is apt to be prevalent occurs more often in cold weather, because people are more likely to be indoors, where air doesn't move and direct contact with germs is likely.

Not all cold viruses strike in cold weather. One family of cold viruses thrives in the summer and brings us the "summer cold." That so-called adenovirus cold is a distant cousin of polio. (Until its eradication by the polio vaccine in the 1950s, polio struck most often in the United States in summertime.)

Why aren't diarrhea and vomiting listed as symptoms of flu?

Typically, flu is an infection of the respiratory system, not the gastro-intestinal tract. Intestinal–or stomach–"flu" is the viral strain that hits without warning like a bomb, consisting of nausea, vomiting, and diarrhea. It is not the same as A-, B-, or C-type flu but is instead a member of the rotavirus family. It is so close in symptoms to various bacterial infections, including forms of food poisoning, that people often misdiagnose themselves.

Gastroenteritis–an inflammation of the gastrointestinal tract–is the more accurate description for this hard-hitting, short-lived germ. It responds well to bismuth subsalicylate, available as Pepto-Bismol. This medicine is known as a microbial because of its success in re-lieving both bacterial and viral forms of this illness. Gastroenteritis can be extremely serious in small children and the frail and elderly because of its dehydrating effects on the body.

Why do I get a fever and chills with the flu?

With flu, we used to think that fevers and chills just came with the ter-ritory: A fever was the elevation of normal body temperature caused by the infection you were fighting. Now, research suggests that fever and chills are not caused by invading viruses; instead, they are symp-toms created by an immune system when it is engaged in a battle to kill or immobilize a virus.

In their studies of the immune system, researchers have con-cluded that fever plays several critical roles in fighting invading viruses. First, viruses thrive at 85°, a cooler environment than normal body temperature provides. A fever's hot environment makes it tough for viruses to reproduce as fast or even survive. Second, your body's immune reaction is a complex, whole-system emergency response that calls upon a variety of lymph cells to produce antibodies to kill or attack the invading germs. New research suggests that these antibodies work much more efficiently in hotter surroundings.

What makes me feel so rotten when I get a cold or the flu?

Like fever and chills, exhaustion and lack of appetite were once considered nonfunctional side effects created by the cold or flu virus. As more research unmasks the inner workings of the immune system response, we are discovering that feeling rotten is the body's way of shutting down everything except essential operations so that all energies can be directed to fighting the invading viruses.

Recent research shows that antibodies called interleukins also trigger the release of hormones that block the body's normal storage of fats and sugars—substances used to produce energy. This puts the body's energy sources at the ready for fueling immune reactions. Temporarily shutting off energy storage and sustaining the immune response take a toll on your energy level and help create the fatigue you feel when you have a cold or the flu.

You may have noticed when you've had a cold or the flu that your muscles seem overly sensitive to pain. Lowering the pain threshold is another action attributed to your immune system. While your joints might not normally ache, they do when your immune response is in high gear. Scientists speculate that the symptom helps ensure you'll slow down and conserve energy needed for waging a successful antiviral battle.

Why do I always hear about the danger of pneumonia with colds and flu? Isn't pneumonia a bacterial disease?

Pneumonia, which refers to inflammation of the bronchial tubes and air sacs of the lungs, is either bacterial or viral. Either type is dangerous, and potentially fatal, especially in young children, those over 65, or in persons with chronic heart, lung or other organ disease, diabetes, or an immune disorder. Pneumonia associated with colds or the flu is called a secondary infection, or a complication. Treatment of bacterial pneumonia, which always requires a doctor's attention, consists generally of a 10-day to two-week course of an antibiotic, such as penicillin, along with plenty of nonalcoholic fluids and rest.

Pneumonia (especially viral pneumonia) can come on so quickly that sometimes it arrives concurrently with the flu or a cold. Viral pneumonia is the most lethal of flu or cold complications because it strikes so quickly and without warning, progresses quickly, and is not bacterial; therefore, antibiotics have no effect on it. Timely treatment is critical, thus it's important to know the classic symptoms of both kinds of pneumonia.

If you have labored or rapid breathing, chest pains (or shortness of breath), wheezing, faintness, shaking chills, or a bad sore throat along with extreme fatigue or irritability, it's important to see your doctor immediately.

In either viral or bacterial pneumonia, look for a fever of at least 101° (especially one that doesn't abate within two to three days) and a cough. Indeed, the type of cough may be your only indicator of whether the condition is viral or bacterial: A cough that raises frequently foul-smelling phlegm of a greenish or brownish color often signals bacterial pneumonia. While viral pneumonia doesn't happen frequently, it may save your life if you know that a *dry, hacking cough that starts at the same time as your fever is often the only indicator of the condition's presence.*

A powerful antiviral drug called amantadine enjoys some success in fighting viral pneumonia, but it works only if administered in the first 20 hours of the disease. Since it can have a range of side effects, it is not widely dispensed, but is used for those most vulnerable to pneumonia fatalities, including the elderly and the chronically ill. A one-time vaccination can protect against pneumococcal pneumonia (but is not effective against all pneumonias). This shot is usually recommended for those in high-risk groups.

What are other complications that follow colds and flu?

Complications are often called masqueraders because their symptoms partially overlap pneumonia characteristics and/or those of other complications. At the outset, what is actually a complication may strike you as "just a persistent cold" or "a bad case of the flu." A good rule of thumb: Colds and flu viruses run the worst of their course within a week. If you have any of the distinguishing symptoms of a particular secondary infection, or if your fever has lingered for more than three or four days, you probably have more than a cold or the flu.

It's important not to let complications get too ingrained before seeking medical attention. (Or if you know you are susceptible to a particular secondary infection, be alert to the first signs of its presence so that medical treatment can start immediately.)

In addition to bacterial and viral pneumonia, here are the most common complications of colds and flu:

■ **Allergic rhinitis (hay fever):** Recurring inflammation and irritation of the lining of the nose and upper respiratory tract as the result of an allergy–a reaction by the body against invasion by a foreign substance the body perceives to be dangerous. Hay fever is usually caused by inhaling an airborne particle contaminated by an allergen. Hay fever does not always accompany or follow colds or flu; it can be a stand-alone condition.

■ **Asthma:** A respiratory condition in which the medium and small air passageways in the head and chest cavity narrow, resulting in breathing difficulties.

■ **Bronchitis:** Inflammation of the air passages of the throat and chest.

■ **Earache:** Bacterial (or sometimes viral) infection, usually of the middle ear, most common in children ages three and under; if not brought under control, this infection can lead to hearing loss and other problems.

■ **Laryngitis:** Inflammation of the voice box, or larynx.

■ **Meningitis:** Severe (bacterial or viral) infection of the membranes covering the brain and spinal cord; can be fatal.

■ **Pharyngitis:** Inflammation of the throat. If bacterial, this is a strep throat.

■ **Sinusitis:** Inflammation and infection of one or more of the sinuses in the face and head.

■ **Strep throat:** Infection of the throat (also sometimes tonsils and adenoids) caused by streptococcus bacteria; can only be firmly diagnosed by throat culture; complications can lead to scarlet fever and kidney problems.

When group A strep bacteria–considered rare by the Centers for Disease Control and Prevention–hit the headlines in spring 1994, it became known as the "deadly flesh-eating bacteria" and the "killer virus" because the bacteria-virus destroyed victims' muscles and either killed them or forced amputation within hours or several days of the onset of the infection. While group A strep is related to strep throat, it does not usually begin as one. Group A strep generally tends to infect a cut or bruise or it may follow a throat infection. Dennis L. Stevens, M.D., at the University of Washington in Seattle, explains: "If you have some sort of trauma, bruise, or injury and you develop a fever, you should be concerned that you have an infection." That's when to seek medical advice. Doctors also warn that group A strep is characterized by *increasing* pain, heat, and redness in the place where you've had a surgical procedure, trauma, or bruise.

Now that you know the working definitions of colds and flu, let's take a look at how to avoid getting them in the first place.

Complications Having Symptoms That May Masquerade As Pneumonia

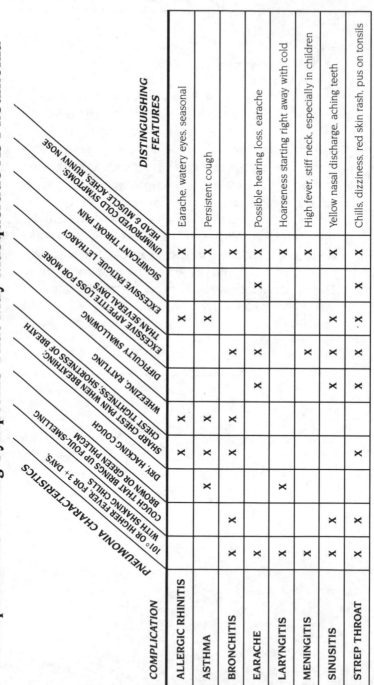

COMPLICATION	101° OR HIGHER FEVER, FOR 3+ DAYS	COUGH THAT BRINGS UP FOUL-SMELLING BROWN OR GREEN PHLEGM, WITH SHAKING CHILLS	DRY, HACKING COUGH	SHARP CHEST PAIN WHEN BREATHING; SHORTNESS OF BREATH	WHEEZING, RATTLING; CHEST TIGHTNESS	DIFFICULTY SWALLOWING	EXCESSIVE APPETITE LOSS FOR MORE THAN SEVERAL DAYS	EXCESSIVE FATIGUE, LETHARGY	SIGNIFICANT THROAT PAIN	UNIMPROVED COLD SYMPTOMS: HEAD & MUSCLE ACHES, RUNNY NOSE	DISTINGUISHING FEATURES
ALLERGIC RHINITIS			X					X		X	Earache, watery eyes, seasonal
ASTHMA			X	X	X			X		X	Persistent cough
BRONCHITIS	X	X	X	X	X					X	
EARACHE	X	X			X		X	X		X	Possible hearing loss, earache
LARYNGITIS	X					X		X	X	X	Hoarseness starting right away with cold
MENINGITIS	X					X	X	X			High fever, stiff neck, especially in children
SINUSITIS	X		X		X		X	X	X	X	Yellow nasal discharge, aching teeth
STREP THROAT	X		X	X		X	X	X	X	X	Chills, dizziness, red skin rash, pus on tonsils

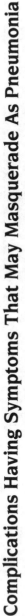

2. Tips on Prevention

Since there are no known cures for colds or flu, prevention must be your goal. A proactive approach to warding off colds and flu, in fact, is apt to make your whole life healthier.

Taking responsibility for your own well-being is a main tenet of the holistic approach to good health. Many prevention techniques come down to using common sense about your health. More and more, medical science is paying attention to the mind-body connection, which has been a staple of Eastern philosophies for centuries. Scientists and doctors are proving increasingly that the mind has a profound effect on the body. Evidence is mounting that strong immune systems are a hallmark for those who have learned to make their lives harmonious and relatively stress free. To achieve this balance takes planning and work, but it can easily become habitual if you decide to make it a priority. Here are specific strategies to employ:

Hygiene

1 Wash your hands.

 Wash your hands often during the day, preferably with a disinfectant, antibacterial soap (such as Dial, Safeguard, or Lever 2000). Remember, however, that washing with plain hot water is better than not washing at all if no soap is available. Wash more frequently if you're around sick people.

Most cold and flu viruses are spread by direct contact and "self-inoculation"—i.e., making yourself sick by touching a virus-contaminated object or person, then touching your eyes, nose or mouth before you wash your hands. Evidence shows that's all it takes. When people with colds or flu who have contaminated hands (from touching their own mucus or phlegm) touch telephones, pens, light switches, water glasses, computer keyboards, or other objects, the germs they leave can live for hours or, in some cases, weeks, only to be picked up by the next person who touches the object.

2 Don't cover your sneezes and coughs with your hands.

Because the germs and viruses cling to your bare hands, muffling coughs and sneezes with your hands results in passing along your germs to others. (Today, experts give more support to direct-contact contagion for most colds; however, a vocal medical contingent supports the aerosol, or airborne, route of contagion for colds and flu, believing that the viruses spread also on contaminated air particles from sneezes or coughs.)

You don't have to be rude by sneezing or coughing directly at someone. When you feel a sneeze or cough coming on, turn your head away or look down while you're expelling your germs into the air. If you find you're instinctively covering up anyway, use a tissue and dispose of it immediately, then wash your hands.

3 Get rid of your cloth handkerchiefs.

Those monogrammed cotton handkerchiefs may be a time-honored family tradition, but using them is a sure way to launch your own personal cold and flu season. These are a loathsome catchall for your germs, as cold and flu viruses thrive in dark, moist environments when the soiled handkerchief is returned to a pocket or a purse. Switch to paper facial tissues instead, and throw them away immediately after using. Be sure to wash your hands once you've blown your nose.

4   Don't touch your face.

Cold and flu viruses enter your body through the eyes, nose, or mouth. Touching their faces with germ-laden hands is the major way children catch colds and flu. All the while mistakenly believing they don't touch their faces, adults travel the same avenue of contagion. In a notable study designed to test how cold germs spread, a University of Wisconsin cold researcher monitored a roomful of adults who had been exposed to cold and flu viruses contaminating objects in the room. He found the average adult touched some part of his or her face 15 or more times an hour, usually without realizing it. Most of those in the room got sick while, in a similar study where participants wore body casts to prevent their hands from reaching the face, significantly fewer caught colds.

5   Use disinfectants at home and work.

Launch an offensive war on germs others carry into your environment. Be especially alert in winter months, when colds and flu are at their peak. Regularly wipe down household and office objects that are frequently touched—telephones, remote control switches, desk or kitchen implements—or those you may be sharing with a cold- or flu-ridden friend or relative. Use Lysol, Pine Sol, or any of the other liquid or spray disinfectants available at the supermarket.

Remember, too, that you're not just cleaning up after others: You can reinfect yourself with your own germs that are left around the house or office.

6   Use paper cups in the bathroom.

Splurge, especially during cold and flu season, and buy a supply of paper cups for the bathroom. Viruses thrive in the bathroom, living for hours or longer on glassware, toothbrushes, and even towels.

7 Don't share your toothbrush.

It's even a good idea to throw out your toothbrush when your cold or flu is over so that you don't reinfect yourself. Since viruses thrive in dark, moist, cool places, damp toothbrushes stored in dark bathroom cabinets are prime storage spots for viruses and breeding grounds for bacteria. So celebrate the end of your cold or flu with a new toothbrush.

8 Change towels often when there's a cold or flu in the house.

Just like toothbrushes, towels and washcloths—especially when damp—harbor live viruses. When you wash soiled cloth towels, use a hot-water wash or one that contains bleach (an antigermicidal) to wash away all of the germs.

9 Keep the sick room healthy.

More than simply a matter of comfort (which goes a long way to helping a sick person feel better), keeping the sick room as clean as possible will prevent you and others from picking up cold and flu germs. Remember to:

■ Change and wash bed linens and bed clothes once a day.

■ Air out the room by opening doors and windows periodically.

■ Rinse oral or anal thermometers in rubbing alcohol after each use.

■ Wipe with disinfectant all lamp and light switches, telephones, remote TV controls, or anything else the sick person or visitors might touch.

■ Empty wastebaskets of dirty facial tissues. Try using plastic liners during a bout with a cold or flu. (Just pinch the plastic bag shut, without having to touch germ-laden contents.)

10 Humidify your surroundings.

The importance of moisture is often underrated as a cold- and flu-fighting tool. Adequate moisture is essential for the proper functioning of mucous membranes, which are the front doors of your upper respiratory system. When a virus enters the nose, hair-like, flagellating cilia mounted on the membrane walls propel it down the sticky, lubricated highway of your nasal passages. Cilia push viruses out of the body by dumping them into the blood's lymphatic "drainage" system where the germs are attacked and immobilized. If the nasal system is dried out due to a lack of adequate humidity, the membrane lubrication disappears and cilia can't function. The breakdown lets invading germs pass through without a fight, and that puts additional requirements on a stronger immune defense.

To adjust humidity in your office or home:

■ Keep relative humidity at a constant, between 50 and 60 percent.

■ Invest in a humidity gauge that measures the air's water content.

■ Add a drum humidifier to your furnace, especially if your home's heat is very dry.

■ Use a portable humidifier in your bedroom or office. Be sure the device is cleaned regularly—preferably daily—so that the water reservoir doesn't harbor bacteria and fungi, which can lead to other infections and allergic reactions.

■ Remember that air-conditioning dehumidifies and can dry you out as much as indoor heating can. Check gauges on window and central air units to see if there's a relative humidity setting. If so, set it at between 50 and 60 percent.

■ Use old-fashioned methods to moisturize a room. Place pans of water around, especially over (or next to) a heat source such as a radiator. (Change water regularly to avoid fungus growth that occurs in standing water.) Add plants to your room or office. Remember your lessons in photosynthesis: Plants need moisture, but in return they give off moisture as an oxygen by-product. (Cacti or other succulents do not count as helpful humidifiers.)

11 Drink plenty of fluids.

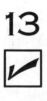 If you want to stay healthy, drink plenty of fluids (water, natural fruit juices, and noncaffeinated herbal drinks) every day. Nearly 75 percent of your body consists of water. Every one of your vital organs needs water to function and survive. Water flushes your system, washing out the poisons as it rehydrates you. A typical, healthy adult needs eight 8-ounce glasses of water or liquids a day. (If 8-ounce portions make you feel like you're drowning, try them in 4-ounce sizes, and schedule "fluid breaks" throughout your day.) One doctor advises his patients that the way to tell if they are drinking enough liquids is to observe their urine color: If the color runs close to clear—instead of a deep yellow—there is probably adequate liquid intake.

12 Use a saline nasal spray.

If you can't affect the humidity around you, affect the moisture level inside your head. Buy a simple, non-medicinal saline nasal spray (available in your local drugstore in a squeeze-and-spray container under such brand names as Ocean or NaSal) and use it several times a day, or whenever your nasal passages feel irritated and dried out. This inexpensive device flushes cold, flu, and dust particles from your nose, while it keeps the mucous membranes moist. A saline spray is especially helpful as a cold and flu preventative on airplanes, where passengers tend to breathe recirculated, dehumidified air.

13 Breathe through your nose, not your mouth.

Breathing through your mouth dries out the mucous membranes in your throat, a line of cold and flu protection you want to have in top working condition. You may not even be aware of how you breathe, so ask a family member or friend to check whether you're a nasal or oral breather.

14 Dab unmedicated petroleum jelly in each nostril.

This is an inexpensive effective antidote to dry nasal passages. Using a dab of petroleum jelly in the morning and again before bedtime will help keep your mucous membranes in fighting shape, and that, in turn, will help repel cold and flu viruses looking for a susceptible host.

15 Take a sauna.

By indulging in a sauna twice a week, you may be able to reduce your susceptibility to colds by up to 50 percent. A 1989 German study showed that those who steamed twice a week got only half as many colds as those who didn't. While not clear on the exact role saunas play in prevention, the researcher postulated that the lower susceptibility rate was probably due to the volunteers inhaling 80° or higher air, a temperature too hot for the cold or flu virus to survive.

16 Be antisocial.

Most cold and flu viruses spread through direct contact with sick people, but some flu viruses and a few of the cold virus strains are known to spread also by sneezing and coughing. High season for colds and flu in a temperate weather zone (which includes much of the United States) is typically November through February. You "shed," or throw off, virus germs that others can "catch" for several days before you come down with symptoms and for up to a week after you've contracted a cold or flu. (The exception is certain flu varieties to which young children are vulnerable which can shed for up to two full weeks *after* flu symptoms have disappeared.) Therefore, you may want to consider restricting your visits to sick friends and family, just as you may want to wait until a week *after* someone you know has finished with a cold or the flu.

If you're in a high-risk health category (suffering from heart, lung, kidney or other chronic diseases; have diabetes or an autoimmune condition; or are 65 or older), be especially careful to shorten (or eliminate) visits with sick friends, especially children (who, because of their daily social contacts in school, their age-limited acquired immunity to illnesses, and their chronically unwashed hands, are known germ reservoirs). If you must visit, sit at a distance, try not to touch objects in the room, and wash your hands immediately after you leave.

17 Get fresh air.

A regular dose of fresh air—to help purge you of any airborne cold or flu viruses—is important, especially in cold weather when central heating dries you out and makes you more vulnerable to cold and flu viruses. During cold weather more people stay indoors, which means more germs are circulating in crowded, dry rooms. By opening windows and doors for a few minutes and circulating fresh air in a room in cold weather, you can help push out airborne viruses. (In summer, fresh air may help to reintroduce humidity into a room that air-conditioning has dried out.)

Immunization

18 Get a flu shot, especially if you're in a high-risk category.

While annual flu shots help protect you against mainly the A- and B-type strains, they enjoy a 75 percent success rate. Unfortunately, since their debut two decades ago, flu shots have been dogged by myth and inaccuracy compelling enough to persuade many people not to take them. Except for those sensitive to eggs (the vaccine is made from killed flu viruses grown on an egg medium, which can cause an allergic reaction in such people), anyone can take the shots. Further, flu shots do not give you the flu. Only a small percentage of complications occurs and is generally limited to chills with fever and headaches (all are immune response reactions, rather than an illness created by the flu vaccine).

Health-care professionals urge annual inoculations for those in high-risk groups, including: those 65 or older; those prone to respiratory diseases; and people who have heart, lung, or other chronic diseases, diabetes, or immunosuppressant disorders. Doctors also advise flu shots for those working in proximity to or with large groups of people or who are institutionalized, since flu spreads by direct and airborne contact and is especially contagious in crowded quarters.

Because certain strains of flu change so frequently, injections are good for only a year and are administered in the autumn, just prior to the start of flu season. They take two weeks to become active. (A split immunization program, with shots two weeks apart, is often administered to children.)

For the record: Flu shots won't keep you from getting a cold, which comes from a different virus.

Diet and Nutrition

19 *Eat healthy.*

☑ Eating right promotes healthy cell and tissue reproduction, maintains strong muscle and bone systems, and provides the body with the fuels it needs to keep the immune system in fighting shape. In 1992 the U.S. Department of Agriculture tossed out its dated wheel of four food groups and replaced it with the five-part Food Guide Pyramid (see page 22). The pyramid's components reflect current thinking about which nutrients are required to keep us healthy, and in what proportions you need to eat them.

20 *Eat your age.*

☑ In 1994 federal law began requiring "Nutrition Facts" labels on all commercial foods. The labels show fat, cholesterol, sodium, fiber, and nutrition contents, serving size, and what percentage its contents represent of an adult's daily calorie allotment. These guidelines, like the FDA food pyramid, are based on a daily 2,000-calorie intake, ideal for an active, younger adult, but too high for the over-50 crowd. (Weight Watchers International suggests that a suitable calorie level for a postmenopausal woman, for instance, is 1,600 calories daily.)

As you get older, the need to eat smarter intensifies. That's when your metabolism slows and you need fewer daily calories but as many or more nutrients. It's vital to get all of the vitamins, minerals, and nutrients you need to keep your immune system in fighting shape to resist colds and flu.

A study reported in the May 11, 1994, *New York Times* identified "the malnourished elderly"–at high risk for flu, colds, and secondary complications–as a large socioeconomic cross section of the over-65 American population. The statistics went on to show that people in the 50-60-year-old group are not eating nutritionally enough either.

To stay healthy, be intentional about what you eat. If you don't know about nutrition or how to tailor daily nutrition plans to your age

Food Guide Pyramid
A Guide to Daily Food Choices

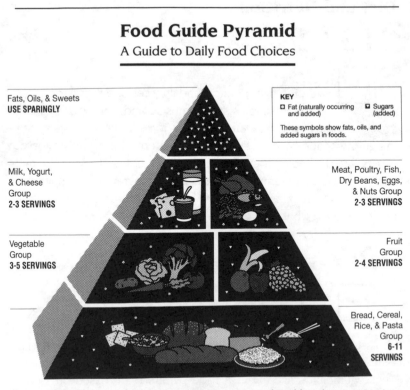

Fats, Oils, & Sweets
USE SPARINGLY

KEY
▢ Fat (naturally occurring and added)   ▨ Sugars (added)

These symbols show fats, oils, and added sugars in foods.

Milk, Yogurt, & Cheese Group
2-3 SERVINGS

Meat, Poultry, Fish, Dry Beans, Eggs, & Nuts Group
2-3 SERVINGS

Vegetable Group
3-5 SERVINGS

Fruit Group
2-4 SERVINGS

Bread, Cereal, Rice, & Pasta Group
6-11 SERVINGS

Source: U.S. Department of Agriculture/U.S. Department of Health and Human Services

and personal health circumstances, numerous learning resources are at your fingertips. Consult your local public library, hospital and college libraries, health reports in daily newspapers, radio and television programs, free lectures at community health services, and call-in telephone help lines.

21 ✔ Practice "genetic nutrition" to keep your immune system in tune.

Help your body fight cold and flu viruses most effectively by limiting foods that are personally bad for you. Medical nutritionists Artemis Simopoulos, M.D., and Victor Herbert, M.D., detail in their book, *Genetic Nutrition**, how each person has a different "genetic blueprint," or diet and nutrition requirements dictated by genetic (inherited) composition and personal environment. They maintain that one, universal, public-health-approved diet is only a start, and may even be harmful to your health, given your personal genetic blueprint. As genetic typing of disease susceptibility comes more into focus, Simopoulos and Herbert argue that, to lead healthier, more disease-free lives, you need to learn about your distinctive genetic and disease heritage, review your current environment, then target those needs in drawing up your individual diet.

22 ✔ Eat foods containing "phytochemicals."

"Phytos" have been making headlines lately: phytotherapy, phytochemicals, phytoingredients. A Greek prefix, "phyto" means plants, and phytochemicals initially referred to the natural compounds in plants that protect them from sunlight. Now, phytochemicals is the umbrella term applied to the array of natural chemical compounds found by the thousands in such whole foods as fruits and vegetables. The latest research, highlighted in the April 25, 1994, *Newsweek*, shows that these substances give virus- and other cold-fighting vitamins in whole foods a supercharged boost. Eating foods containing phytochemicals contributes to your everyday health, and

*New York: MacMillan, 1993.

some also help prevent more serious disease. Here are some of the phytos you'll be hearing more about:

■ **Sulforaphane:** A tumor-blocking substance found in broccoli, cauliflower, brussels sprouts, and kale.

■ **Allylic sulfides:** Found in garlic and onions. These validate the ancient claim that garlic is an excellent natural preventative for colds, flu, other infectious diseases, and chronic conditions such as stomach cancer.

■ **Flavonoids** (or **bioflavonoids**): Found in green plants, citrus fruits, and berries such as currants. These exponentially boost vitamin C absorption in the body, thereby fortifying the immune system against colds and flu. They are now also thought to block cancer-causing hormones from latching onto a cell.

23 Eat yogurt.

Eating a daily cup of low-fat yogurt can put a crimp in your susceptibility to colds and flu. A 1991 study at the University of California (Davis) School of Medicine found that yogurt-eaters have a 25 percent reduced susceptibility to colds. Researchers also noted that, of those who got colds, the yogurt-eaters got rid of their cold symptoms faster than the non-yogurt-eaters. The scientific explanation? Researchers believe that yogurt's active cultures—beneficial live bacteria (labeled "live" or "active" on the yogurt label)—enter the body and stimulate production of immune system substances that fight disease.

24 Eat garlic.

Tales of the medicinal powers of garlic have been around virtually for ages: The herb has been used as a preventative and curative since pre-Biblical times. More and more, garlic is looking like the all-purpose wonder herb. In addition to being one of nature's most effective immune system stimulants that fends off colds and flu, there's evidence that garlic helps lower blood pressure, thin blood, lower serum cholesterol levels, and aid digestion. In his book, *Prescription for Nutritional Healing**, natural food author Jerry Balch reports on microbiology studies at Brigham Young University that pinpoint garlic's ability to destroy certain viruses associated with the common cold and at least one version of the flu.

When eaten, the garlic component called allium (an amino acid derivative) changes to allicin, a natural antibiotic, capable of anti-bacterial action equivalent to 1 percent of penicillin. (It was used to treat wounds and infections in World War I.) For those who don't want to ingest whole garlic on a daily basis, it's now available in an odorless supplement form, although eating the whole food in raw form may pack more of an anti-cold and -flu punch. Raw garlic contains more than 200 phytochemical compounds that humans have not yet been able to replicate totally in pill form.

25 Reap the benefits of immune-boosting herbals and botanicals.

Health-giving foods and tonics made from plants and trees have been used for centuries. While many natural concoctions are used to relieve cold and flu symptoms (see Chapter 3), a number are considered health-boosting preventatives good for everyday use. Here are a just a few:

■ **Ginger:** Used in teas and cooking to induce sweating and ward off colds; also, to settle upset stomachs caused by flu or motion sickness; root and powdered forms. To make a tea, steep a pinch each of powdered ginger, peppermint, and clove in a cup of boiling water.

■ **Ginseng:** Steeped in teas; root, tincture, and powdered forms. A mild stimulant, it contains stomach-settling ingredients and an array of vitamins that fortify the immune system, and provides an energy boost.

■ **Kelp:** Used as a salt replacement in main dishes, this seaweed is often used in powdered form and is a rich source of vitamins and trace minerals.

---

*Garden City Park, N.Y.: Avery, 1990.

■ **Reishi (shitake) mushrooms:** Used in a variety of main dishes; dry or powdered forms. Helpful for building resistance to viral infection, they contain a virus that stimulates interferon production.

■ **Royal jelly:** A honey and pollen derivative, especially high in the B vitamins. This substance also contains vitamins A, C, D, E, and an array of minerals and amino acids. Boosts the immune system.

Check with your library for books on herbals and botanicals or locate a health food store for more information.

Vitamins and Minerals

26 *Include vitamins and minerals in your cold- and flu-fighting artillery.*

The 13 organic substances known as vitamins required to regulate the functioning of cells and the 13-plus chemical elements called minerals that must be present in the diet to maintain good health have long been the province more of alternative health disciplines than the medical establishment. Since the first vitamin was isolated in 1911, science has struggled to pinpoint the exact role vitamins and minerals play in cellular and immune functions.

A 1968 World Health Organization report contained some of the first scientific evidence linking adequate dosages of vitamins and trace minerals with resistance to colds, flu, and other infections. Only two years later, Nobel laureate Linus Pauling, Ph.D., galvanized health-conscious Americans by extolling the near-miracle properties of vitamin C, which he advocated taking in large daily doses as a cold preventative. By the late 1980s, scientists had discovered antioxidant qualities of vitamins–their ability to rid the body of harmful "free radical" cells that, left unchecked, diminish the immune responses and cause cancer and other life-threatening or fatal illnesses.

By the mid-1990s, the cavalcade of new discoveries about the legitimate role of vitamins and minerals in preventing illness has placed these natural elements on the new frontier of biomedical research, not to mention on the dinner plate and in the medicine cabinet.

27 *Try vitamin C.*

Does it or doesn't it help prevent colds and flu? After decades of research, a consensus has emerged from the health community that says this leading antioxidant is vital to cellular health and immunity. Vitamin C stimulates the production of interferon, a natural virus killer, and mobilizes the immune cells that roam the body to attack invading cold and flu viruses. While there's still disagreement in the health community as to whether vitamin C prevents colds and flu, there is nearly universal acceptance that this vitamin can spare you many bouts with colds and flu and make them shorter when you do have them.

Since 1970, when Linus Pauling advised people to take a gram or more of vitamin C a day to reduce colds by a frequency of 45 percent, debate has continued over the proper daily amount. There is no right answer: The federal Recommended Dietary Allowance (RDA) for vitamin C suggests a daily maximum of 60 milligrams, but RDAs were created to establish the minimum amount of a vitamin or mineral needed to avoid a deficiency; hence, RDAs typically are low dosages. Then, too, some leading cold researchers discounted early clinical trials showing vitamin C's ineffectiveness as a preventative because they felt 250 mg./day was too small to be significant.

At the other extreme, large-dose proponents are led by Pauling followers and natural medicine practitioners who call for 3,000-5,000 mg. (3-5 grams) daily as a cold preventative. The answer is somewhere between the extremes, probably 250-1,000 mg. daily when you are well. We suggest you experiment with what's right for you, keeping the following in mind:

■ Vitamin C is a strong acid, so it's best not to take it in supplement form (pills or liquid) on an empty stomach.

■ The healthiest way to ingest vitamin C is to eat it in natural foods —citrus fruits, tomatoes, and green vegetables—because then you'll be benefiting also from the natural compounds called bioflavonoids. These boost the effectiveness of vitamin C and aid its absorption by the body.

■ Vitamin C is destroyed by heat, so uncooked fruits and vegetables are best.

■ Megadosing with vitamin C produces a toxic reaction in the form of stomach pains and diarrhea. In some, it may lead to kidney stones, a good reason to check with your doctor about what an effective and safe dose for you might be.

28 Add zinc to your diet.

☑ Successfully resisting colds and flu depends on an immune system that's in top shape. The mineral zinc is critical to your immune system's health because it helps initiate antibody production and is active in the circulation of disease-fighting T-cells. Studies show that, in animals and humans alike, resistance to cold and flu viruses and secondary infections of the respiratory tract is impossible if there is a zinc deficiency.

Researchers have noticed that zinc is commonly deficient in many of us and especially lacking (by as much as 50 percent of the RDA) in older people. The good news is, zinc doesn't take long after it's ingested to have a positive effect.

The RDA for men is 15 mg., for women 12 mg. Find small but adequate amounts of zinc in wheat germ, meat, whole grains, and seafood, especially oysters and crabmeat. If you can't reach your RDA by eating whole foods, zinc supplements come in lozenge and pill form. Don't megadose. Taking too much zinc over long periods of time can be detrimental to your HDL (the "good" cholesterol) and trigger other reactions that eventually can lead to heart disease and thyroid problems.

29 Review whether you're getting these other immune-boosting and antioxidant vitamins in your daily diet.

☑ According to the U.S. Department of Agriculture, at least a third of Americans consume less than 70 percent of the RDA of vitamins A and C, and the B-complex vitamins, as well as the minerals calcium, iron, magnesium, and zinc. In addition to vitamin C and zinc, there are other important vitamins and minerals needed to help prevent catching a cold or flu. (RDAs for 25-50-year-old women and men appear in parentheses.)

■ **Vitamin A:** Essential to immune system stimulation and production of the substance that lines the respiratory tract. Deficiency weakens these membranes. Beta carotene, a vitamin A derivative, helps increase disease-fighting T-cells. Without vitamin A, cilia "slough" off and cells lose their ability to secrete mucus; consequently, mucus doesn't trap or propel cold or flu viruses entering the nasal passages. Mucus also contains lysozyme, an enzyme that destroys microbes, including viruses. (women: 8,000 I.U.; men: 10,000 I.U.)

■ **The B-complex vitamins:**

- **thiamin** (B_1): helps cells convert carbohydrates into energy (women: 1.0-1.1 mg.; men: 1.2-1.5 mg.)

- **riboflavin** (B_2): helps cells convert carbohydrates into energy and is essential for red blood cell growth (women: 1.2-1.3 mg.; men: 1.4-1.7 mg.)

- **niacin** (B_3): aids in the release of energy from foods and helps maintain healthy skin (13-19 mg.)

- **pantothenic acid:** vital for food metabolism and the production of essential body chemicals; helps adrenal function and antibody formation (no RDA available; experts recommend 4-7 mg./day)

- **pyridoxine** (B_6): aids in chemical reactions of proteins and amino acids, and in forming red blood cells (women: 1.6 mg.; men: 2.0 mg.)

- **biotin:** expedites the metabolism of protein, carbohydrates, and fat (no RDA available; experts recommend 30-100 mcg./day)

- **folic acid:** important in normal cell growth, protein metabolism; deficiency decreases T- and B-cell functions, immunoglobulin secretions, and phagocytic activity of the neutrophils, all vital internal immune responses to cold and flu invasions (women: 180 mcg.; men: 200 mcg.)

■ **The mineral iron:** A deficiency in this mineral causes immune dysfunctions, including shrinking of lymphatic tissues, defective functioning of several disease-fighting substances, and fewer fighter T-cells. (women: 10-18 mg.; men: 10 mg.).

Other important vitamins in your diet include B_{12}, central to red blood cell production (2 mcg./day); and antioxidants D, which helps maintain blood levels of calcium and phosphorus (5 mcg. or 200 I.U./day), and E, which helps form red blood cells and may improve immune functions in older people (women: 8 mg.; men: 10 mg.).

If you're eating regular, nutritious meals, you may be getting the full RDA of many of these vitamins and minerals in your food. If not, often just adding a good multivitamin to your daily regimen will be all that it takes. Megadosing is not recommended; it may even be harmful.

30 Reach your vitamin quota by eating whole foods.

In search of the quick fix and the magic pill to offset harried schedules where nutritious meals may be overlooked, Americans have hit the vitamin stores with fervency this last decade—one that saw new discoveries unfolding about the natural disease-preventing and immune-boosting prowess of vitamins and minerals. (A 1994 article in Newsweek reported that in 1993 we spent $123 million buying vitamin E, a 39 percent increase over the year prior, and $117 million on vitamin C, up 10 percent over 1992.) But do pills offer what whole food can't?

The main message from the phytochemical frontier is: No vitamin pill by itself has been proven to give the super boost to the body that vitamins in their natural forms do. So, whenever it's possible, go for the real thing.

Lifestyle

31 Don't smoke.

Statistics show that heavy smokers get more severe colds and more frequent ones.

Smoking and being around tobacco smoke profoundly zap the immune system. Scientists think that inhaling tobacco smoke makes a person more vulnerable to catching colds, flu, and related complications and makes colds last longer because the smoke dries out and paralyzes cilia. These are the delicate hairs that line the mucous membranes and, with their wavy movements, serve as brooms that sweep cold and flu germs out of the nasal passages. Once cilia break down permanently (inevitable in heavy smokers, but likely in anyone who is around smoke on a regular basis), germs enter the respiratory openings more freely, raising susceptibility to colds and flu. Experts contend that one cigarette can paralyze cilia for as long as 30 to 40 minutes.

32 *Cut alcohol consumption.*

Forget the old saw about alcohol being good for a cold because it sterilizes the germs out of existence. The two are not fellow travelers: Alcohol enters and leaves the body through the gastrointestinal system, while colds and flu viruses travel almost exclusively in the upper respiratory tract. Moreover, alcohol is a depressant that slows bodily responses to your environment and diminishes your ability to get rid of invading cold, flu, and other viruses.

Heavy alcohol use destroys the liver, the body's primary filtering system, which means that cold and flu germs won't leave your body as fast. The result is, heavier drinkers are more prone to initial infections as well as secondary complications. Even in moderate doses—up to 4 ounces a day—alcohol dehydrates the body. For every ounce added, alcohol takes more fluids from the system, also depleting the essential A, B, and C vitamins (the antioxidants, so vital to maintaining the healthy functioning of the immune system).

33 *Reduce your caffeine intake.*

Duke University scientists have recently found that stress-related hormones are considerably higher in coffee drinkers, compared to those who drink a placebo. "Caffeine interacts with stress and intensifies it," says James Lane, a professor of psychiatry at Duke University. If you down a lot of coffee or tea a day, eat quantities of chocolate, or drink a variety of carbonated sodas, you're getting an infusion of caffeine. Along with increasing stress and anxiety levels (neither of which is good for fighting colds and flu), caffeine dehydrates the body, which leaves you receptive to cold and flu infections.

34 Sleep to beat colds and flu.

It may not be a peculiarly American trait to burn the candle at both ends, but dozens of sleep studies indicate that we as a nation are desperately sleep-deprived. Most of us cheat ourselves of at least one to two hours of sleep nightly—out of the seven to nine hours of rest per night the studies say we need. As sleep debt accumulates, it lowers the effectiveness of your immune response to cold and flu germs. Sleep is the principal activity that revitalizes cells and recharges your vital organs, your muscles, and your ability to think clearly. So make it a habit to meet your needed sleep quota.

35 Create and maintain as pollution-free an environment in your home as possible.

Chemical pollutants harm your body in different ways. Pollutants damage and diminish your immune response to colds and flu, making you more susceptible to invading viruses. Indeed, our very homes can be major sources of pollution. In poorly ventilated houses, stale air that contains fumes, smoke, and dust can be a health problem.

Don't buy heavy-duty chemical solutions for cleaning and maintenance, when more natural cleaners—such as household ammonia—will do. Buy only small quantities of paints and hydrocarbon solvents: paint thinners, upholstery cleaners, lighter fluid, and the like. Use them sparingly and be certain to ventilate the areas where you use them. Favor pumps over aerosol sprays of most household products.

36 Beware of pollution at work.

No job is totally pollution-free, of course. Remember, though, that air, chemical, and water pollution all work against your immune system. Bad air and chemicals paralyze your upper respiratory system defenses, which in turn allows cold and flu viruses easier entry into the body.

Whether you're already employed, looking to change jobs, or are on the job hunt, be alert to the same types of pollutants that you're keeping out of your home—cleaning supplies, solvents, and other chemical compounds. If your present or prospective office is not legally a nonsmoking area, work to make it smoke-free. Also, ventilate your work area with fresh air whenever possible.

Stress

37 Reduce stress to keep colds and flu at bay.

Stress consists of the external demands placed on you and your internal reaction to them. While a natural part of life, stress can get out of hand; when it does, you live in a state of high anxiety, panic, or depression, and are at your most susceptible, studies repeatedly suggest, for catching a cold or the flu. Unfortunately, stress is not easy to dodge in our complex society.

Reducing stress, which allows the immune system to fight colds and flu more effectively, is a learned response, explains psychologist James Mills, Ph.D., who, in his book *Coping With Stress**, recommends lowering the stress level by acquiring 12 stressbusting skills. Mills suggests that, if you're deficient in any of them, you write down the step(s) and a schedule for mastering each skill. To reduce stress, learn to:

■ tolerate uncertainty

■ anticipate change

---

*New York: John Wiley & Sons, 1982.

- develop competencies

- satisfy wants (within reason)

- resolve conflicts in your life

- clarify your values (to yourself, then to others)

- reduce demands on yourself

- assume control of your life (even in small pieces)

- reduce uncertainty

- finish unfinished business

- minimize change

- seek support

For a quick stress reducer: Release tension in your shoulders by "dropping them down" until you feel the muscles around your neck, shoulders, and upper back go slack. Then breathe in until your chest swells. Now exhale. Repeat three or four times until you feel the anxiety seep out of your body.

38 *Relax.*

If you teach yourself how to relax, you can activate your immune system on demand. There's evidence that when you put your relaxation skills into action, your interleukins – leaders in the immune system response against cold and flu viruses – increase in the bloodstream immediately. Start by training yourself to picture an image that you find pleasant or calming. If your mind wanders, force it back to the image. Do this exercise 30 minutes a day for several months. "Relaxation is a learnable skill," says researcher William H. Keppel, M.D. But it's different strokes for different folks, he adds, noting that some people equate thinking about happy events with relaxation, while others summon thoughts about positive feelings. If you encounter a mental block, you may want to learn how to relax by taking up yoga or t'ai chi, forms of meditative exercise we'll discuss later.

39 Learn the difference between relaxation and "doing nothing."

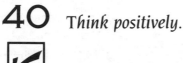

Relaxing—by concentrating on a happy memory, an activity you love, a place you dream of traveling, or a person who makes you feel good about yourself—stimulates the part of your brain that increases disease-fighting hormones in the body. But don't confuse this active daydreaming with inactivity or trying to concentrate on an activity that bores you silly. A recent study checked blood samples of the relaxed and the bored and found that, when participants are genuinely relaxed, disease-fighting hormones showed up in the blood within minutes. However, for those in the bored and inactive groups there was no significant change in blood chemicals.

Attitude

40 Think positively.

Studies show that the brain's positive thought patterns stimulate release of cold- and flu-busting interleukins. Bad or negative emotions set off a very different chain reaction than positive feelings, often releasing substances that depress your immune responses.

Researchers believe that an optimistic view of life's situations has much to do with how and whether the body releases endorphins, the hormones that ameliorate pain (in the case of colds and flu, the discomfort of symptoms). One convincing study of the positive-mind/well-body connection involved 141 students facing deadlines. Conducted by researchers at Carnegie-Mellon University and the University of Miami, the study found that those who were more optimistic reported fewer headaches, stomach problems, cases of depression, and other symptoms than their downcast associates.

41 Don't worry yourself sick.

Living with anxiety and stress for any length of time helps set the stage for you to catch colds, flu, or other illnesses. When a person is under extreme or continuous stress, the blood is flooded with adrenaline and other stress-response chemicals that activate the "fight or flight" response. If you're on perpetual alert, your stress-response chemicals accumulate and can lead to mental and emotional problems, while making your immune system less effective for warding off everyday germs. Interestingly, among other damaging effects attributed to the fight-or-flight stance are congested nasal passages, which researchers believe directly contribute to lower resistance to colds and flu.

In a 1992 study reported in American Health, a group of 400 volunteers—some under heavy stress, others without any—were given germ-filled nasal drops. Researchers found the stressed volunteers twice as likely to develop colds. The findings of noted cold researcher and psychologist Sheldon Cohen, Ph.D., of Carnegie-Mellon University, indicate that stress stimulates hormones that may suppress your immune cell function. Subsequent studies show that a high-stress period often exactly coincides with the 24-to-72-hour incubation period for a cold.

When you can't seem to stop worrying, isolate your worries by writing them down on paper. Then break each concern into smaller parts. Look at what's on the list that you can change and note how. Make a realistic schedule for starting to change what you can. Look at what you can't control. Ask yourself what is the worst that can happen if you can't change something. Look at these as challenges rather than as insurmountable obstacles. Then put the challenges into a mental "compartment" that you'll deal with later and concentrate on living in the present.

42 Laugh away colds and flu.

There's mounting evidence that those who harbor anger and hostility are more vulnerable to all kinds of illness, from colds and flu to chronic and life-threatening conditions. No one understands clearly why laughter is the best medicine, but doctors credit hearty laughter with the same health-giving positive effects that aerobic exercise provides: increased heart, respiratory and circulation rates. And, like exercise, laughter stimulates the release of endorphins –the opiate-like hormones that kill pain, make us feel good, and help alleviate depression. It's no coincidence that quite a few hospitals and medical centers are currently studying the link between laughter and self-healing. Laughter is healthy for everybody. And those who laugh a lot have a hard time staying angry.

43 Make friends.

People who have support systems in their families, spouse, friends, business, and/or social organizations live a life "outside of themselves." Those who are isolated–by choice or circumstances–develop more colds and cases of flu with worse symptoms than their socially tuned-in peers. Research, including studies done at England's Common Cold Research Unit, supports the notion that loners get colds as well as more serious diseases more often–and for longer duration–than their "connected" peers. As to why this occurs, one theory centers on the depression that often accompanies loneliness. Depression decreases the body's disease-fighting immunoglobulin, and that, in turn, makes a person especially susceptible to any cold or flu virus that comes along.

44 Schedule rewards and happy times in your life.

Permitting yourself to take "pleasure breaks" as a part of your routine will help keep your immune system in tip-top shape and help you avoid contracting colds and flu. If you're in the middle of a stressful situation, schedule a time-out to visit with a good friend. Escape reality for two hours by going to or renting a movie you've been wanting to see. Read a favorite author or play a set of tennis with those friends who make you laugh.

Findings reported in 1994 by State University of New York at Stony Brook psychologist Arthur Stone, Ph.D., showed that those people who reward themselves by doing something pleasurable can count on an immune system boost that lasts for a couple of days. Contrarily, the immune systems of those confronted with a day of unrelenting bad stress showed immediate negative effects.

45 Schedule work breaks and vacations.

Health studies show that people are happier, more productive, and healthier when they take regular work breaks from whatever it is they are doing. Changes of scenery, pace, and activity refresh your mind and body while giving your immune system the boost it gets whenever you are enjoying yourself.

46 Aim for balance in your life.

Yin and yang, work and pleasure, diversity, balance. Good balance—where all of your self-esteem and happiness are not wrapped up in one aspect of your life, whether social, work- or family-related—is healthy. An imbalance, in which you invest all your time and psychic energy in only one dimension of your life, exposes you to anxiety and depression when something goes wrong. Irritability, defensiveness, and isolation can easily follow, all of which have negative effects on the immune system.

Exercise

47 Do aerobic exercise regularly to keep your immune system in top condition.

Exercise is essential to health, and aerobics are essential to exercise. Aerobic exercise speeds up the heart to pump larger quantities of blood; makes you breathe faster to help effect oxygen transfer from your lungs to your blood; and makes you sweat once your body heats up. Exercise is aerobic when your body's cells develop the ability to extract larger amounts of oxygen from the blood; the heart becomes larger and more efficient at pumping; and the cells collect oxygen more easily.

These exercises help relieve stress (by getting rid of excess adrenaline) and depression (by triggering release of endorphins). They also tone your muscles, strengthen the bones, and keep the immune system vital. A California State University study reported in the June 1994 *Men's Health* found that just 30 minutes of aerobic activity has an immediate effect of reducing body tension and releasing blood substances that boost your immune system. A Loma Linda University study reported in the January 1993 *Redbook* found that exercising for 20 to 40 minutes two to four times a week helps increase the body's natural virus-killing cells.

Aerobics are a workout, but they don't have to include jumping and landing, which may be tough on your knees and other joints. New studies show that even moderate exercise is helpful and healthy. Whatever you do, it is important to first consult with your practitioner about your goals and type of workout.

48 Try acupressure exercises if you can't do aerobics.

If arthritis or other painful motion-limiting conditions are keeping you from the exercise routines that will fortify your immune system, you may want to turn to acupressure exercises. Acupressure identifies pain-relief points throughout the body that you can activate or stimulate by applying finger pressure.

Acupressure, like its first cousin acupuncture, establishes nerve points, or "meridian" lines, throughout the body, through which life's energy is thought to flow. Proponents of the technique suggest that applying pressure to strategic nerve points influences your body to release endorphins into your bloodstream, which then desensitize pain and encourage relaxation.

Acupressure exercises can be helpful and stress-relieving, especially for those who may live with chronic pain or limited range of motion. Michael Reed Gach's book, *Arthritis Relief at Your Fingertips**, is an excellent source of acupressure exercises. If you suffer from

---

*New York: Warner Books, 1989.

arthritis or another motion-limiting condition, check with your doctor before starting an acupressure–or any–exercise regimen.

49 Train your body and your mind using meditative movement therapy.

Meditation or meditative exercise–achieving inward concentration that allows you to clear the mind of thoughts and focus on your senses–is a form of learned relaxation that stimulates endorphin release into the bloodstream and antibody production. Meditative movement therapies such as yoga and t'ai chi are not only good exercise programs (excellent for those who do not like jarring exercises), but their meditative components raise the conscious mind to a different level, thereby helping eliminate stress.

■ **T'ai chi** (also called t'ai chi ch'uan) centers on the same fundamental principle as other Chinese therapies, that to harmonize the body forces encourages life's energy (chi) to flow. Often called meditation in action, this exercise therapy consists of slow, well-ordered, deliberate movements that promote physical strength, mental clarity, and emotional serenity. Although gentle and serene in its routines, t'ai chi leads practitioners through exercises demanding the full range of motion.

■ **Yoga** is a mind-body therapy that combines prescribed postural poses with breathing exercises and specific, measured body movements. The Americanized version of this Indian movement therapy is now practiced by some 3-5 million Americans. Yoga provides physical and mental benefits, and pain and stress relief.

3 Tips on Treating Colds and Flu

Americans spent in excess of $2.3 billion in 1993 on more than 300 nonprescription cold and flu treatments. With no cures in sight for cold or flu viruses, treatments can at best bring relief, lighter symptoms, or a shortened duration.

Most cold and flu drugs are broad-spectrum applications that ameliorate symptoms rather than attack specific viruses. Cold and flu medical treatments fall into five categories: analgesics; antihistamines; cough remedies; decongestants and nasal inhalants; and anesthetizing respiratory remedies.

While there's no cure, there's also no one right way to treat a cold or a case of flu. That leaves the relief picture wide open to a myriad of remedies, from home-based to those requiring medical attention. Here are tips from a variety of sources for alleviating cold and flu:

50 Know when *not* to treat symptoms.

Research shows that your symptoms, not the invading cold or flu virus, cause you to feel sick. Far from being symbolic and nonfunctional (as was thought until recent studies reversed thinking), symptoms are part of the healing process—evidence that the immune system is battling illness. Consequently, the current approach to cold or flu treatment is not to medicate a symptom, unless it's absolutely necessary.

To illustrate, a fever not only warns us that we're seriously sick with flu or another kind of infection but it's also evidence that your body is trying to kill viruses in a hotter-than-normal environment (viruses thrive at 85° or lower). And a fever's hot environment makes germ-killing blood proteins circulate more quickly and effectively. Thus, says the new thinking, you should probably endure fever's discomfort for a day or two rather than lower it with an antipyretic/analgesic—an action that may have the accidental effect of making your flu or cold last longer. (It bears mentioning that research has found that aspirin not only lowers a fever but also makes you more contagious by significantly increasing the number of viral particles you "shed" in mucous secretions.)

Recent studies by Johns Hopkins University researchers found that analgesics actually can depress the immune system. Doctors are starting to believe that *not* taking analgesics may make a cold or flu run its course more quickly, while also killing off invading viruses more completely. (Remember the fever clues that signal a secondary infection: a 101° or higher fever for three days or more, or higher than 101° at the outset. Don't even think about medicating yourself under these conditions. Call your doctor right away.)

Similarly, productive coughing is nature's way of clearing breathing passages from accumulating phlegm—the thick mucus of a cold or flu that traps germs and moves them to the lymph glands or other clearing systems of the body. By taking a cough suppressant, you may be quashing a helpful recuperative tool: More and more experts believe it's better not to treat "productive coughing."

Nasal congestion is another symptom best treated mildly or not at all. A decongestant clears blocked nasal passages by restricting the flow in blood vessels to the nose and throat. However, say doctors, often you *want* the increased flow because it warms the infected area and helps secretions escort the germs out of your body.

Drugs

51 See which over-the-counter (OTC) drugs might be appropriate, when treating a cold or flu.

Many medicines began as prescription-only remedies, usually sold at much higher prices, before they were available in OTC forms. The Food and Drug Administration (FDA) has lifted many prescription-only boundaries as soon as the efficacy of the medication has been proven.

Surveys estimate that some 60 percent of the time, Americans self-treat their colds and flu (not always efficaciously, perhaps) using nonprescription drugs. Talk with your doctor or pharmacist about effective substitutions for prescription drugs.

52 Buy store brand relief.

When purchasing OTC drugs in your drugstore or super-market, select store brand labels. Stores buy these drugs in bulk and sell them under their own brand name or label—usually at a cheaper price. The drugs generally have the identical active ingredients and are as effective as brand name medications. Learn to compare labels for active ingredient equivalencies and contents.

53 Take analgesics to relieve pain and/or lower your fever, if your discomfort is extreme.

We know we've said it's better not to medicate cold or flu symptoms. But we also know there are times when a fever or muscle aches may make you too uncomfortable to get much-needed rest. If you must medicate for fever pain, use an OTC analgesic judiciously. Analgesics are drugs that desensitize you to pain, and they also have antipyretic, or fever-lowering, qualities. Aspirin, acetaminophen, and ibuprofen—each available over-the-counter—are the most frequently used analgesics for relieving cold and flu muscle aches and pain.

Aspirin and ibuprofen block the body's production of prosta-glandin, the substance released when you suffer an injury that triggers signals to the brain to feel pain, while acetaminophen blocks pain impulses in the brain itself.

Here's a closer look at the three main choices in analgesics:

■ **Aspirin (acetylsalicylic acid):** *Relief action*: Reduces inflammation, fever, pain. *Form(s)*: Straight, compound, or buffered (the latter helps lessen stomach irritation). *Typical brands*: Bayer, Anacin (undiluted), Bufferin, Empirin, Ascriptin (buffered with antacids), Excedrin (combined with acetaminophen). *Adult dosage*: Typically two 5-grain (300 mg.) tablets every 3-4 hours as required. *Possible side effects*: May irritate stomach lining, cause nausea, pain, occasionally a peptic ulcer, ringing in ears; can bring on internal bleeding in those who cannot tolerate it; not given to those approaching surgery because it is an anticoagulant; long-term overuse can damage kidneys. Aspirin should not be given to children or young adults (16 and under) as flu or cold treatment due to their susceptibility to Reye's syndrome.

■ **Acetaminophen:** *Relief action*: Reduces fever and pain, but does not affect inflammation. *Form(s)*: Tablet or liquid (the latter generally for children). *Typical brands*: Tylenol, Datril, Liquiprin, Tempra. *Adult dosage*: Same as aspirin, two 5-grain tablets every 3-4 hours. *Possible side effects*: Long-term overuse can damage liver, especially if taken in combination with alcohol.

■ **Ibuprofen:** *Relief action*: Reduces fever, muscle pain, inflammation. *Form(s)*: Tablets. *Typical brands*: Advil, Nuprin, Motrin. *Adult dosage*: Usually two 200-mg. tablets, every 3-4 hours; maximum recommended daily intake is 1,200 mg., although prescription strength is generally much stronger. *Possible side effects*: May irritate stomach lining, causing stomach bleeding (less toxic to stomach than aspirin, more toxic than acetaminophen); long-term overuse in large doses can sometimes lead to kidney problems.

Allergic reactions to one or more of the analgesics is possible, and those allergic to aspirin may also be allergic to ibuprofen. In all cases, but especially if you suffer from any chronic diseases of the heart, kidney, stomach, or lung, check with your doctor before you self-medicate.

54 Avoid the shotgun approach to relieving nasal congestion.

Multi-ingredient cold remedies often try to relieve all cold and flu symptoms, so it's not unusual to see decongestant and antihistamine ingredients aimed at relieving nasal congestion, runny nose, sneezing, and itchy or watery eyes. A number of these multi-symptom treatments come in a timed-release form. But cold research experts counsel against what they call a "shotgun approach" of using one formula to bring relief to multiple symptoms.

"The trouble with multi-symptom cold medicines is there's not enough dosage to adequately relieve each individual symptom," says Ellen O'Connor, M.D., of Thomas Jefferson Medical University in Philadelphia. "They also tend to have a lot of extra ingredients you don't need, such as alcohol or caffeine." As an example, some liquid cold formulas contain 25 percent alcohol—twice the percentage of alcohol found in most wines and more than half that of 80-proof liquor.

Doctors point also to timed-release medicines that offer too low a dosage at the timed intervals to be most effective. Then, too, some brands contain combinations that work at cross purposes: a multi-ingredient cold remedy that fights drowsiness while promoting sleep. Or a combination cough remedy that advertises it will suppress coughs *and* expectorate cough-producing mucus.

Doctors recommend instead that you target a single-focus medication to relieve your most uncomfortable cold or flu symptom—for example, an analgesic if your muscles ache.

55 Use a decongestant to relieve nasal congestion.

Decongestants relieve nasal stuffiness and improve breathing. A decongestant's active ingredient stimulates a narrowing of infection-swollen blood vessels in the sinuses and membranes that line the nose, thus reducing swelling and inflammation, which in turn eases breathing. Unlike antihistamines, decongestants do not dry up nasal secretions but rather decrease the amount of mucus produced by the nasal lining.

Decongestants come in pills and liquids (oral) and drops or sprays (topical). Oral decongestants are systemic—they affect your whole body—and can raise your blood pressure. With their stimulant action, oral decongestants can also produce restlessness and insomnia. Read labels first and know if there are any limits on what you can take. Those who take medications for depression, those with high blood pressure or heart disease, and those who are or who have been treated for prostate cancer are warned against taking decongestants.

The Public Citizen's Health Research Group (PCHRG), in its book, *Worst Pills, Best Pills II**, which reviews and rates drugs, recommends against oral decongestants because "they contain large amounts of amphetamine-like drugs that can increase heart rate and blood pressure." However, it does note that the FDA has reviewed what it feels are three safe and effective oral decongestant ingredients, contained in the products Afrinol, Actifed, Sudafed, and a variety of prescription cold and cough drugs.

PCHRG advises cold and flu sufferers to favor topical decongestant nose drops or sprays: "You get 1/25th as much of these drugs just in the nose, where needed, instead of throughout your body." The group strongly cautions users to follow instructions.

56 Limit use of a nasal spray to three days.

 The upside to OTC nasal inhalants is they work fast and locally to open breathing passages. The downside is, using them for more than three days in a row is likely to start a "rebound infection," causing congestion that outlasts the cold and possibly creating a dependency on the nasal inhalant.

If you're wondering how it's possible to become addicted so quickly, health writer Michael Castleman, in the February 1989 *Saint Raphael's Better Health Letter*, explains how the rebound condition typically occurs: After three days of being contracted (by application of the spray, which helps constrict the swollen capillaries that cause congestion), the tiny muscles in the nasopharynx become fatigued, stop

---

*Washington, D.C.: Public Citizen's Health Research Group, 1993.

responding to the spray, and become more swollen than they were to begin with. The only way to reopen nasal breathing passages under rebound conditions is to reuse the nasal inhalant. Doctors report many cases of having to wean patients off nasal inhalants that have been used for too long.

PCHRG recommends nose drops or spray containing oxymetazoline hydrochloride (Afrin, for example), xylometazoline hydrochloride (4 Way Long-Acting Spray), henylephrine hydrochloride (Neo-Synephrine nasal spray or nose drops), or their generic equivalent.

57 Don't take antihistamines for colds or flu.

Antihistamines are drugs that block the effects of histamines—the natural chemicals (antibodies) released by the body during an allergic reaction. Antihistamines do relieve the watery eyes, runny nose, and itchy palate of hay fever, but studies show they have little positive effect on the nasal congestion of rhinovirus colds. Double-blind studies in 1987 showed that nasal symptoms and mucus production did not differ among rhinovirus-inoculated groups given antihistamines and placebos.

The use of antihistamines as a palliative for colds or flu can carry a double negative: They dry out the mucous membranes (just when the immune response is relying upon mucus to carry invading viruses through the lymph and other clearing systems) and can cause drowsiness. Antihistamines may actually encourage mucus to thicken and slow down (as it dries out), adding to your congestion and eventually leading to a cough. And their side effects can include dizziness, loss of appetite, dry mouth, nausea, blurred vision, and/or difficulty passing urine.

Antihistamine-based cold formulas aimed at relieving nasal congestion and providing cough control often advertise that their ingredients will dry out mucous secretions as well as suppress the brain's nerve impulses that control coughing. But as we've already pointed out, if you're letting your immune response run at full throttle to kill your virus most efficiently, you won't want to be treating more than one symptom at a time. So go for a less medicating, more direct approach —a cough remedy for a cough or a decongestant for congestion.

58 Use cough medicines sparingly and wisely.

Coughing is one of the mechanisms the lungs use to clear themselves of invading particles such as viruses, bacteria, and inhaled smoke. The mucus that normally lines the lung walls thickens with immune secretions when you have a cold or flu. This mucilaginous—or gluelike—substance helps the body trap invading germs so they can be propelled out of the airways by hair-like cilia. The result is expectorating—coughing up or bringing up thickened, virus-filled mucus.

A cough that brings up phlegm or sputum is a "good cough," known as a productive cough. Rather than medicate, the best thing you can do to help a productive cough is drink water-based warm or hot liquids (natural expectorants) to thin mucus (allowing you to expectorate it more easily) and keep fluid in your respiratory tract.

By contrast, a nonproductive cough is dry and hacking, with no mucus, the kind that accompanies many colds and the flu. Since this cough is not beneficial to clearing the lungs, doctors are more apt to suggest a cough remedy for this condition, especially so the patient can sleep. For nonproductive coughs, try a cough suppressant, or antitussive. PCHRG recommends using suppressants with dextromethorphan (Hold, St. Joseph's Cough Syrup for Children, Sucrets Cough Control Formula). If you absolutely must take a cough medication, try to avoid alcohol-based cough suppressants or those containing anesthetizing narcotics—such as codeine—since each can be addictive. Also, the use of narcotics often leads to constipation.

59 Use anesthetizing lozenges and gargles for temporary relief of a sore throat.

When you're looking for sore throat relief, sucking on a menthol-, benzocaine-, or phenol-based lozenge may be your most effective choice. In addition to keeping the throat moist, these lozenges help numb the throat, while giving you a feeling of more wide-open nasal passages. Be sure to follow dosage directions. Lozenges are medicines, too, and overuse of their ingredients can backfire and irritate your already sore throat.

No lozenge or throat treatment brings more than a respite. The FDA Advisory Panel considers the following active ingredients safe and effective for reducing sore throat irritation:

- benzocaine (Children's Chloraseptic, Spec-T Sore Throat Anesthetic Lozenges)

- hexylresorcinol (Sucrets)

- menthol (Luden's Menthol Lozenges)

- phenol and sodium phenolate compounds (Cherry and Menthol Chloraseptic Lozenges, Cēpastat)

Commercial mouthwashes and gargles containing phenol and sodium phenolate (Chloraseptic and Cherry Chloraseptic Liquid and Aerosol Spray) can provide temporary relief from sore-throat pain. Neither these nor other mouthwashes or gargles possess germicidal properties that prevent a cold or flu, however, nor do they provide a cure, in spite of active ingredients that imply otherwise, says the FDA panel of experts.

Finally, advises the panel, avoid aspirin-containing chewing gum for sore throat relief. Their tests found insufficient evidence that topically used aspirin relieved throat pain (they caution that it may even irritate inflamed mucous membranes).

Medical Attention

6O *Don't let sore throat relief mask a strep throat.*

If you're using medicine to relieve the pain of a sore throat, be careful that you're not masking signs of a strep throat, the secondary bacterial infection that can escalate into rheumatic fever, earache, or meningitis if not caught in time and medicated properly. Strep infections are especially common in children and often difficult to diagnose as being different from a regular sore throat.

Be familiar with the key symptoms of a strep throat, which we detailed in Chapter 1. When a sore throat persists and meets the criteria for strep, settle it with a throat culture.

61 Ask your doctor to prescribe amantadine to reduce Type A flu effects, if you're in a high-risk health category.

If you experience lung, heart, or other chronic diseases; are 65 or over; or live or work in a nursing home or other institutional environment—and you missed flu shots for the year and now have flu symptoms—you may be a candidate for the prescription antiviral drug amantadine hydrochloride. Taken in the first 20-48 hours that symptoms appear, the medicine usually shortens and reduces impact of Type A flu, says John R. LaMontagne, Ph.D., of the National Institute of Allergy and Infectious Diseases. "It can cut in half the number of days you suffer from fever and other flu symptoms," he says, noting that even starting the drug as late as day three of the flu lessens the disease's effects. Amantadine does carry the risk of side effects, especially in the elderly. Five to 10 percent of those who take it experience nausea, lightheaded-ness, and/or insomnia, reports the National Institutes of Health.

62 Don't take antibiotics for a cold or flu, unless you and your doctor know you have a second-ary infection such as sinusitis or strep throat.

Antibiotics have no effect against viruses, so they are ineffective as cold or flu treatments. Yet many of us pressure doctors into prescribing them anyway.

"Forty to 60 percent of all antibiotics in the United States are misprescribed," says Sidney M. Wolfe, M.D., director of Public Citizen's Health Research Group. Further, today a number of serious bacterial infections have grown resistant to penicillin and other broad-spectrum antibiotics. In early 1994 the Centers for Disease Control and Prevention (CDC) reported that 28 percent of children with ear infections were resistant to penicillin and broad-spectrum antibiotics. Consequently, the group called upon doctors to be extremely judicious in prescribing antibiotics.

The CDC also advised individuals to purge their medicine cabinets of old medicines. Leftover or outdated prescriptions are not necessarily the right ones to kill your present virus, even if you have a bacterial complication, because a partial prescription works only part way.

63 Treat sinus infections early.

Until recently a sinus infection, or sinusitis, was always thought to follow colds or flu as a bacterial complication. Now, research led by cold expert Jack M. Gwaltney Jr., M.D., of the University of Virginia Medical Center, provides evidence that some sinus infections start concurrently with the viral infection. Reporting in the January 1994 *New England Journal of Medicine*, Gwaltney identified early onset inflammation of one or more of the sinus cavities as a "co-infection." The findings promise to rewrite cold and flu lore.

If you're one of the 30 million Americans prone to sinus infections, don't wait until your cold or flu begins to abate to confer with your doctor if symptoms of a secondary infection have appeared. Call immediately once you identify these sinusitis hallmarks: nasal congestion, plus a headache with pain or pressure around the face; excessively sensitive upper teeth; and/or yellow or green nasal drainage. Sinus infections that get deeply ingrained before you start a course of antibiotics are more difficult to cure and present the additional danger of evolving into other, potentially more serious complications such as bronchitis or pneumonia.

64 Ask for a doctor's appointment in the morning.

The morning is rush hour for nasal mucus, when head congestion from a cold, flu, or a secondary infection is at its worst. Concentrations of plasma proteins—key components of nasal membrane inflammation—were tested around the clock in cold-ridden volunteers by a Swedish researcher, who discovered that concentrations at 4 a.m. and 8 a.m. were five and 20 times higher than at 4 p.m. So if you want to be certain your doctor sees all of your symptoms, most likely at their worst, choose a morning appointment.

Home Remedies

65 *Blow your nose often (and the right way).*

✔

It's important to rid your nasal passages routinely of mucus buildup when you have a cold or flu rather than sniffling it back into your head, which can complicate matters by creating ear congestion. But careful—the harder you blow, the better the chance that pressure created by the blowing will force germ-carrying phlegm back into the ear passages. This can lead to an earache in addition to the cold or flu you already have. The best way to blow your nose: Press a finger over one nostril while you blow *gently* to clear the other.

Remember that cold or flu nasal congestion is always at its worst first thing in the morning. If trying to blow your nose when you first awake is futile, wait until you've "been vertical" for a few minutes. Typically, phlegm and mucus begin to break up once your body emerges from its prone sleep position.

66 *Use a bulb syringe filled with warm salt water, if your congestion is higher up in the nasal passages.*

✔

Here's a popular antidote for breaking through nasal congestion: Mix ¼ teaspoon salt and ¼ teaspoon baking soda in 8 ounces of warm (or warmer, not hot) water. Use a bulb syringe to squirt water into the nose. Hold one nostril closed by applying light finger pressure while squirting the salt mixture into the other nostril. Let it drain. Repeat 2-3 times, then treat the other nostril. Repeat several times daily. Or use a store-bought saline spray.

Salt-water rinsing helps break up local mucous congestion while it removes dust and virus particles and bacteria from your nose before your cold gets more serious. (Don't share your syringe or spray, and wash it with hot water between dosings.)

67 Try these time-tested home remedies for colds and flu.

■ **Drink chicken soup.** Whether it's the steam, the thickness, or the memories of childhood you associate with it, chicken soup really does help clear the nasal clog. Some researchers speculate that the viscous properties of your grandmother's best-loved cold remedy slow the rush of neutrophils to the site of a flu or cold infection–the cause of congestion and inflammation. Others feel its steam humidifies and acts as a decongestant. Irwin Ziment, M.D., professor of pulmonary medicine at UCLA, offers author Jean Carper a slightly different version in *Food: Your Miracle Medicine**: A protein containing the natural amino acid cysteine is released in the soup, and cysteine thins the mucus in the lungs, thereby breaking up congestion.

■ **Stay warm.** A chill doesn't directly cause a cold. On the other hand, staying warm when you're down with a cold or flu helps your body direct its energy reserves toward the immune battle rather than toward stoking up your personal furnace to protect you against cold.

■ **Rest.** The battle waged by the immune system the first few days of a cold or flu taxes the body. Let your body's energy reserves help the immune system do its work by giving in (whenever you can) to the fatigue that accompanies your illness.

■ **Gargle.** Gargling–tilting your head back and swishing a liquid around at the back of your throat–can be tried with a variety of mixtures to moisten a sore throat and bring temporary relief.

■ Try a teaspoon of salt dissolved in warm water, four times daily.

■ Take an astringent gargle–made with tea that contains tannin–to tighten the membranes and reduce the tickle in your throat.

■ Use a thick, viscous–or mucilaginous–gargle, popular in folk medicine lore: One tablespoon dried raspberry leaves (available at your local health food store), two cups boiling water, one teaspoon honey. Let leaves steep in boiling water for 10 minutes; strain; add honey. Cool to room temperature. Gargle at full strength. (Can be stored up to three days in a refrigerated, airtight container.)

---

*New York: HarperCollins, 1993.

■ **Drink hot liquids to relieve nasal congestion, prevent dehydration, and soothe inflamed membranes.** According to flu expert James Pascal Imperato, M.D., cold liquids impede mucus and can contribute to congestion. Hot drinks, on the other hand, help loosen secretions that might otherwise settle in and contribute to a secondary, bacterial infection. Sipping a hot toddy before bed to clear a stuffy nose and promote sleep is an age-old remedy. Here's an easy recipe: Into a cup of steaming hot herbal tea mix one teaspoon of honey and one shot (1½-2 ounces) of whiskey or bourbon. Limit yourself to one, though. Too much alcohol inflames the mucous membranes and produces a counterproductive effect. A nonalcoholic old favorite for soothing a sore throat and cutting bronchial phlegm is plain, hot tea with honey. Remember that many teas contain caffeine, which you should use in moderation or not at all when you're sick.

■ **Drink fluids until your urine runs clear.** When a fever causes the body to dehydrate and lose vital salts, you may think you are rehydrating more than you are. You need to drink at least eight 8-ounce glasses of liquid a day, preferably more when you have a cold or the flu. If your urine is a bright yellow, you have not yet consumed enough liquids.

■ **Take a sponge bath.** Use lukewarm, not cold or hot, water to soothe and relax you, while reintroducing moisture to your skin.

■ **Take a steamy shower.** It reintroduces moisture to your body (and your nasal membranes) and is relaxing. If you're dizzy, try running a steamy shower while you sit elsewhere in the bathroom to do your sponge bath.

■ **Inhale steam.** Bring a pot of water to a boil. Remove from heat. "Tent" a towel over your head, bend over the steaming water (being careful to avoid steam burns), and inhale. The steam dilutes mucus and helps it drain while producing a soothing effect on your irritated nasal and throat tissues. Add a dab of mentholated salve, if you like. Or use a drop of eucalyptus, pine, rosemary or thyme oil (four cups boiling water to three to four drops oil). Breathe in vapor for 10 minutes. Repeat two to three times daily.

■ **Use a vaporizer or a humidifier.** Rooms low in humidity are your enemy when you have a cold or the flu. You should introduce some means of humidification into your bedroom, especially in winter. Whatever device you use, be fastidious about cleaning it daily, using a diluted bleach mix, then rinsing thoroughly. The water reservoirs of such devices, if left to stand, spawn mold and bacterial growths, which will add to your breathing problems rather than help them.

■ **Use a salve under your nose.** Nose Better is a commercial product containing camphor, lanolin, eucalyptus, and vitamin E. Or try Vicks VapoRub or another mentholated salve to open breathing passages and help restore the irritated skin at the base of the nose. Menthol, eucalyptus, and camphor all have mild numbing ingredients that should help relieve the pain of a nose rubbed raw.

■ **Rub a mentholated salve on your chest.** A menthol or camphor rub on your chest when you're suffering from a cold or the flu can be comforting and may help you breathe better at night. Be sure to cover up, since menthol stimulates the nerve endings that register cold and, even used in a warm room, can make you more susceptible to chills. (Chest rubs with a medicated salve are not always suitable treatments for children, for whom the medication may be too strong and produce skin irritation.)

■ **Apply hot or cold packs around your infected sinuses.** Either temperature works. Decide which feels better on you. Use damp washcloths heated for 55 seconds in the microwave (test temperature for personal preference), hot towels (heated in the clothes dryer), or a hot water bottle. Reusable hot and cold packs are commercially available. Heat them on the stove in hot water (usually for 10 minutes) or in a microwave (30 seconds to two minutes) or place them in the freezer (30 minutes to one hour).

■ **Sleep with an extra pillow under your head at night to help drain upper respiratory congestion.** If the angle is too awkward for sleeping, try placing the pillow(s) between the mattress and your box spring to create a more gradual slope.

■ **Get a massage from a family member or friend.** A massage will relax you, dispel cold and flu aches and pains, and trigger a release of endorphins (the hormones that make you feel good) into your system.

■ **Eat proteins.** Flu and associated fevers cause a breakdown of body cells, reminds James Pascal Imperato, M.D., in his classic book, *What to Do About the Flu**. Your body needs protein-containing

---

*New York: E.P. Dutton, 1976.

foods to rebuild those cells and to get you over the weakness you experience with the flu.

68 Know what's myth and what's fact.

Myths by definition have been around for awhile, may contain a grain of truth, and die slowly if they die at all. Here's an update on 10 that should no longer be considered 100 percent gospel truth:

■ *Myth: Cold weather causes colds and flu.* Many studies over many years, starting earlier in this century at England's Common Cold Research Unit, show that weather has little direct effect on causing colds and flu. As we mentioned already, cold weather contributes indirectly to the cold and flu statistics because it usually forces people indoors into dry, heated areas, where viruses, especially airborne flu viruses, spread and contaminate faster. Research reported in the January 29, 1990, *U.S. News & World Report* found that when one person in a family has a cold or the flu, every other family member has a 40 percent chance of catching it.

■ *Myth: Don't go outside with wet hair; stay out of drafts; stay warm in winter.* Even after years of trying to make the link, evidence is inconclusive that any of these three actions cause one to catch a cold or the flu. A famous British experiment conducted more than 50 years ago drenched volunteers with water, then put them in the way of cold drafts. They fared no worse than those who stayed warm and dry. The same type of study has been repeated in various settings, with the same results. End of myth?

Noted cold researcher Elliott Dick, M.D., points to studies showing that chilled animals contract pneumonia easier. So, while there's no conclusive evidence establishing these three admonitions as fact, each may contain enough common sense to hold your attention.

■ *Myth: Keep your feet warm and dry to avoid colds and flu.* The late British cold expert Christopher Howard Andrewes, who founded the Common Cold Research Unit, exposed volunteers to drafty halls and cold foot baths and found no ill effects. Prevailing theory still holds that you need to come in contact with a cold or flu virus to catch it.

■ **Myth**: *Wear a hat in winter so you don't catch cold or the flu.* No direct link has been proved. However, it's a fact that a majority of your body's heat loss in cold air is through an uncovered head. If you are fighting other infections or are stressed-out and run-down, getting chilled can draw off valuable immune-fighting energies to warm you up. In that case, wearing a hat in winter may not be a bad idea, but not wearing one won't give you a cold or the flu.

■ **Myth**: *Commercial steam-inhaling machines will cure your cold.* In 1989, soon after they were first marketed, these commercial devices that resemble small hair dryers and blow medicated hot air up your nose, were subjected to rigorous clinical scientific review. Studies found conclusive evidence that the devices did not cure a cold. Results as to whether the devices were beneficial in reducing symptoms were inconclusive. In other words, using a towel tent over a steamy, menthol-medicated pan of steaming hot water may produce the same relief for less money.

■ **Myth**: *Kissing spreads colds.* One study showed that it took 1,000 times more rhinoviruses to give someone a cold if a contaminated solution dripped on the tongue instead of the nose. The reason is probably that cold and flu viruses prefer the hotter environment of the nose to the mouth. (But a gallant suitor should think twice before kissing the hand of a cold-infected love. The hand is a much more certain route of germ transmission, since rhinovirus spreads most efficiently through direct, rather than airborne, contact.) Kissing cold-infected friends does carry a warning: At least one cold virus—the adenovirus—is known to spread by oral contact.

■ **Myth**: *Suppressing a cough causes pneumonia.* Not true, reports leading cold researcher Jack M. Gwaltney, M.D., of the University of Virginia Medical Center. "This is a danger only for those with chronic lung disease, such as emphysema, not for normal healthy people with a cold." If the cough is productive, keep coughing. If the cough is dry and hacking, on the other hand, take a single-ingredient cough remedy, especially if you are missing sleep at the expense of your cough.

■ **Myth**: *Starve a fever, feed a cold.* Or is it the other way around? It doesn't matter if you can never remember, because it's a myth. Modern theorists point out that fever often makes a person feel nauseated, so there's a natural tendency to starve a fever. Further, feeding a cold has no scientific basis. Medical practitioners would rather see you drink plenty of liquids (hot or cold) for cold relief.

■ *Myth: Don't exercise, or you'll get sicker.* Common sense should put the kibosh on vigorous exercise when you have a cold or the flu. And you don't want to do any exercise when you have a fever, for fear, among other good reasons, of running your already high body temperature up into the heat exhaustion zone, warns Bryant Stamford, Ph.D., of the University of Louisville School of Medicine. Once the fever is past, milder exercise like brisk walking for up to 30 minutes at a clip is beneficial for getting the white blood cells (and thus antibodies) circulating.

■ *Myth: Cola syrup stops nausea.* Studies show that this age-old home remedy does not settle the stomach in any significant way. Very often, say medical researchers, cola syrup intensifies the nausea of a cold- or flu-related upset stomach because of the mixture's heavy syrup content. As a stopping agent for vomiting, however, this favorite home remedy's heavy sugary syrups may have the effect of relaxing an agitated stomach.

Vitamin, Mineral and Food Remedies

69 *Take (more) vitamin C.*

Much has been said about the dosage of vitamin C recommended once a cold or flu sets in. At one extreme was Nobel laureate and vitamin C champion Linus Pauling, who admitted to ingesting upwards of 20 grams (20,000 mg.) a day when beset by a cold or the flu. But the more modest regimen Pauling advocated for others in his book *Vitamin C and the Common Cold** still applies: "When a cold does start, you should take 500-1,000 mg. every hour for several hours, or 4-10 grams (4,000-10,000 mg.) daily if the symptoms don't disappear with lesser amounts."

Vitamin C boosts the immune function by stimulating production of the natural virus killer, interferon, and mobility of the substances that directly attack invading viruses. According to the December 1989

*San Francisco: W.H. Freeman, 1970.

Whole Foods, studies show that if you take it in combination with bioflavonoids (phytochemicals found just under the rind in citrus fruits, among other places), vitamin C gets a boost that can reduce the duration of a cold or the flu by as much as 50 percent.

Augmenting vitamin C when you have a cold or flu gains support from leading cold researcher Elliott Dick, M.D., of the University of Wisconsin, whose study in the 1980s found that cold sufferers taking 500 mg. of vitamin C four times a day had only half as many symptoms as those not taking vitamin C at all. (In three separate 1991 trials, Dick found that vitamin C did not prevent infection but "markedly, consistently, and significantly reduced signs and symptoms of rhinovirus colds," he told *American Health* in 1993.)

Since vitamin C is an acid, multiple grams of it may not appeal to you or sit well with your stomach. (Effects of overdosing vary from individual to individual and include diarrhea, nausea, and/or stomach pains.) But it's important to take enough to make a difference: Researchers suggest that several clinical studies on the effects of vitamin C were inconclusive because volunteers took too few milligrams (under 250 mg./day) to count.

70 Try taking zinc gluconate lozenges.

Taking the mineral zinc almost immediately stimulates antibody and T-cell production and helps fuel circulation of the white blood cells that rid the body of cold and flu viruses. In 1984 University of Texas researchers conducted clinical studies in which people with common colds dissolved a 23-mg. zinc lozenge or a matched placebo in the mouth every two wakeful hours. After seven days, 86 percent of the zinc-taking subjects were free of cold symptoms, compared to only 46 percent of the placebo-treated subjects. They concluded that zinc lozenges shortened the average duration of common colds by about a week.*

Not all zinc lozenge experiments have had the same good results, however. One conducted at the University of Pennsylvania and

---

*Feltman, John, ed. *Prevention's How-To Dictionary of Healing Remedies and Techniques.* Emmaus, Pa.: Rodale, 1992.

another, carried out in 1987 by cold researcher Jack M. Gwaltney Jr., M.D., at the University of Virginia Medical Center, showed that zinc lozenges had no pronounced beneficial effects on shortening the cold's duration.

Zinc does have a significant effect on strengthening the immune system, however. A new study by Ananda S. Prasad, M.D., of Wayne State University School of Medicine, reported in the March 23, 1994, *Star-Ledger*, focused on 118 healthy 50-to-80-year-olds. The 30 percent who had zinc deficiencies also had lower immunity.

A word of caution: Prolonged zinc overdosing can lead to cholesterol, heart, and thyroid problems. Opinion on how much zinc is too much is divided, so we suggest that, if you're thinking about taking zinc lozenges, you seek your doctor's recommendations.

71 *Adjust your vitamins when you have a cold or flu.*

Studies show that increasing vitamin and mineral supplements when you have a cold or flu can have some positive results. The added vitamin and mineral punch may help shorten duration and severity of your illness. There are many schools of thought concerning which in particular to augment.

Here's a vitamin diet, adjusted for an adult with a cold or flu, recommended by James F. Balch, M.D., in *Prescription for Nutritional Healing**. He advises reducing the normal food diet and increasing fluid intake. Then, he says, take the following daily doses of supplements:

■ **Vitamin A:** 15,000 I.U. plus 15,000 I.U. of beta carotene (to help heal inflamed mucous membranes and strengthen the immune system);

■ **Vitamin C:** 5,000-10,000 mg., in divided doses (to destroy cold viruses);

■ **Zinc gluconate lozenges:** Dissolve one under the tongue every three hours during the first three days of a cold or flu, then drop to one every four hours for a week.

---

*Garden City Park, N.Y.: Avery, 1990.

... ...a that whole foods, especially ...getables, contain thousands of natural disease-fighting compounds called phytochemicals that boost the efficacy of the food's vitamin contents. In *Food: Your Miracle Medicine*, Carper reviews everyday foods that help you get well when you have a cold or the flu. In its April 25, 1994, issue, *Newsweek* published an in-depth look at the world of phytochemical research, citing common foods that contain miracle compounds that help you get rid of viruses. Here are highlights of foods associated with colds and flu:

■ **bananas and plantains:** Soothe upset stomach, strengthen stomach lining against acid; antibiotic.

■ **bell peppers:** Help immune system fight colds, asthma, bronchitis, respiratory infections; high in vitamin C.

■ **blueberry:** Blocks the attachment of bacteria-causing chemicals; curbs diarrhea; antiviral activity; high in natural aspirin.

■ **cabbage and cauliflower:** Cruciferous vegetables with antiviral powers; well-known antioxidants, abundant in numerous strong phytochemical compounds.

■ **carrot:** Immune-boosting, infection-fighting antioxidant containing beta carotene.

■ **chili peppers:** Antibacterials, antioxidants; open sinuses, air passages, break up mucus in lungs; expectorants and decongestants; prevent bronchitis; phytochemical properties from capsaicin, the compound that makes peppers hot. Painkillers, alleviate headaches

immune function.

■ **mustard (including horseradish):** Decongestant/expectorant, breaks up mucus in air passages. Remedy for congestion caused by colds, sinus problems.

■ **onion (including shallots, yellow, red, not white):** Powerful anti-inflammatory, antiviral, antioxidant with strong phytochemical sedative; fights asthma, chronic bronchitis, infections.

■ **pineapple:** Antiviral among other healing attributes; has enzyme that suppresses inflammation.

■ **plum:** Antiviral, laxative.

■ **raspberry:** Antiviral, high in natural aspirin.

■ **rice:** Antidiarrheal.

■ **seaweed (kelp):** Antiviral that boosts immune functioning; high in iodine, so some people may have reactions to it.

■ **soybean:** Active antiviral agent.

■ **strawberry:** Antiviral.

■ **tea (including black, oolong, and green, but not herbals):** Ingredient catechin makes it antibiotic, antidiarrheal, antiviral; ingredient caffeine makes it diuretic, analgesic, and a mild sedative.

■ **turmeric:** Anti-inflammatory agent on par with cortisone; studies show it reduces inflammation in animals, and arthritis symptoms in humans; boosts stomach defenses against acid.

■ **yogurt:** Boosts immune response, spurs activity of killer cells that attack viruses; a cupful daily reduces colds, other upper respiratory infections (URI) in humans; helps prevent, cure diarrhea.

Herbal and Botanical Remedies

73 *Reap the benefits of herbal and botanical relief.*

"Herbs were the original medicines," writes Michael Castleman in *Cold Cures**. "Herbs were typically dried before they were used medicinally; the word *drug* comes from the German word *droge*, which means 'to dry.'" Herbs and other natural remedies have been called the templates for modern medicine: Some 25 percent of our conventional drugs originate from plants and trees. Even more pharmacy products mimic (synthesize artificially) or contain the pharmacological active component of the plant. Aspirin is one of the most prominent medications with herbal roots. Acetylsalicylic acid—aspirin's scientific name—is synthetic salicin, a derivative of the bark of the white willow tree.

"The interest in herbal products is at an all-time high," Purdue University professor Varro E. Tyler, Ph.D., an expert in pharmacognosy (the study of drugs from natural sources), told the *Star-Ledger*. "Interest has been spurred by the disillusionment of medicine—that it can't cure everything and it's costly." Not everyone uses herbals as medicinal replacements; some make good supplements. Check with a qualified practitioner to be sure the herbals you're planning to take are not working at cross purposes with any other medication you may be taking or, in combination, giving you too strong a dose.

Buy herbals and botanicals in health food stores, through mail order, and in some supermarkets. Herbal preparations are not regulated by the FDA, but in 1990 the agency published a list categorizing herbals and botanicals into three groups: *safe and effective; safe;* and *do not use.*

Remember that just because herbals and botanicals are natural and unregulated does not mean they can't be harmful. Before you use them, ask and read about them, then carefully follow instructions on

---

*New York: Fawcett Columbine Books, 1987.

their use. Be especially alert to rare but potentially potent side effects; for instance, herbals are not recommended for those with hay fever or other plant allergies. People with high blood pressure are warned against certain herbals that can raise blood pressure, so be sure to check first.

During a cold or case of flu, Michael T. Murray, D.N., author of *Encyclopedia of Natural Medicine**, suggests taking botanicals three times daily in any of the forms noted below. The equivalencies are:

■ Dried root (as a tea): 1-2 grams

■ Freeze-dried root: 500-1,000 mg.

■ Tincture (dilution of 1:5): 1-1½ teaspoons

■ Fluid extract (dilution of 1:1): ¼-½ teaspoon

■ Powdered solid extract (dilution of 4:1): 250-500 mg.

A sample of medicinal herbs used in cold and flu remedies appears in the box on pages 66-67.

Self-Care

74 *Curtail bad habits.*

When you've come down with a cold or the flu, avoid bad habits or taxing activities that irritate your body, namely:

■ **Don't smoke or breathe in tobacco smoke around you.**

■ **Avoid alcohol** (except maybe for a hot toddy before bed). Alcohol causes mucous membranes to swell, adding to your congestion; it depresses your immune system; it dehydrates you; and it can depress you.

■ **Avoid fatty foods.** Digesting heavy fats taxes your system and takes energy away from the battle being fought by your immune system.

■ **Don't be a workaholic.** First, you may be shedding viruses (up to at least three days into your cold and sometimes 10 days or more after your first flu symptom appears), so you're exposing friends and colleagues to your active germs. Second, when your body's energy

---

*Rocklin, Ca.: Prima, 1991.

reserves are distracted from an all-out immune response, it may take you longer to shake your bug–or may push it into a secondary infection because your resistance is low. Finally, several recent studies have shown that powers of concentration–and sometimes physical coordination–plummet with colds and flu, making you less productive and attentive.

75 Use acupressure to relieve muscle aches associated with colds and flu.

Acupressure, the therapy used to stimulate the body's energies at precise points using the finger and thumb, can be a relief-giving process for cold and flu aches and pains. In his book Arthritis Relief at Your Fingertips*, Acupressure Institute of America Director Michael Reed Gach discusses acupressure points that relieve discomfort from colds, fever, chest congestion, bronchitis, sore throats, coughs, headache, and runny nose. For example: "To relieve fever, colds, flu, and depression in addition to general aches and pains," he writes, "locate the body's Point #5, just below the elbow joint, at the outer end of the crease where your arm bends. At this point, use your thumb to press deeply into the elbow joint, while partially flexing your arm."

Norman C. Shealy, M.D., director of the Shealy Institute for Comprehensive Health Care in Springfield, Missouri, offers this acupressure treatment for a cold- or flu-related (nonmigraine) headache: "Place the tips of your two index fingers at the base of your skull. Move fingers out to either side, until you feel painful, tense little notches. When you locate the spots, press hard. In several seconds, you should begin to feel relief. Reapply pressure for relief. If this fails, press hard on the web of skin between your thumb and forefinger." †

76 Don't fly unless necessary when you have a cold or flu.

There's no point in adding stress to your already stressed-out upper respiratory system, and that's what the change in air pressure will do. Flying with cold or flu congestion

---

*New York: Warner Books, 1989.
† Feltman, Prevention's How-To Dictionary.

Sampling of Botanicals Used for Cold and Flu Relief

BOTANICAL AND FAMILIAR NAME (LATIN NAME)	DESCRIPTION AND PARTS USED IN TREATMENT	COLD AND FLU RELIEF PROPERTIES AND METHODS OF USE
Echinacea Purple Coneflower *Echinacea augustifolia*	Hairy 1- to 5-foot tall perennial herb native to North America with purple flowers, lance-shaped leaves. Root.	Enhances variety of immune functions, decreases infectivity of invading organisms; increases production, activity of interferon; analgesic; relieves nasal congestion. Root extracts made into tea used as antiviral in flu relief.
Chinese Ephedra Mahuang *Ephedra sinica*	Many-branched, broomlike shrub with yellow-green flowers; native to China. American relative is Mormon tea. Branches, stems, bark.	Significant bronchial dilator (decongestant), stems are source of ephedrine used for relief of colds, coughs, asthma. Synthesized ingredient, pseudo-ephedrine, is major component of commercial decongestants. FDA allows up to 1% ephedrine in OTC cold remedies. Those with heart conditions should not take. Herb often used in tea form by Chinese. A stimulant, it may cause insomnia.
Eucalyptus Blue Gum or Fever Tree *Eucalyptus globulus*	Giant (300 feet) evergreen from myrtle family with tall, straight, smooth gray trunk, leathery blue-green leaves, native of Australia but now found in warmer climes of North America. Fresh leaves to make oil; dried leaves are aromatic.	Aromatic oil is ingredient of many commercial preparations used to clear mucus from nose, lungs, lymph system. Steam inhalations relieve coughs; salve used to open nasal passageways, bring relief to chest congestion. Oil used in some cough drops, syrups. FDA allows 1.3% in cough suppres-sants. Used in tea to relieve coughs. Oil's strength may cause choking or skin irritation in children.

porarily damage your eardrums as a result of pressure changes
takeoff and landing. If you must fly, use a decongestant and
a nasal spray with you for use just before takeoff and landing.
ing gum and swallowing frequently also help relieve pressure.

77

Use this relief-by-symptom reminder list the next time you have a cold or the flu.

In addition to recommendations made earlier in this chapter that have across-the-board application in cold d flu relief treatments, here are suggestions and reminders specific these cold or flu symptoms:

■ **aches and pains:** For discomfort take analgesics (children 6 and under should use acetaminophen to avoid contracting Reye's syndrome); try acupressure, massage, herbals containing capsaicin (such as cayenne mixtures), ginger, or garlic.

■ **appetite, loss of:** Drink juices, bland hot soups until appetite returns. Don't force solids too soon. Then move to bland foods (plain toast with jelly, consommé, boiled vegetables, chicken) to give nutrients and needed salts.

■ **chest, tightness or pain in:** Rule out pneumonia by cross-checking your symptoms with pneumonia characteristics (see page 9); try chest rub with mentholated salve, followed by steamy shower.

■ **chills:** Increase fluid intake (dehydration aggravates chills); layer clothing so you can easily dress up or dress down to accommodate body temperature; take herbal remedies that are ginger-based or capsaicin (hot pepper)-based.

■ **cough, dry:** Rule out viral pneumonia; drink fluids; suck on lozenges; gargle; if losing sleep due to cough, try cough suppressant; try mucilage-containing herbal remedies that coat throat for relief.

■ **cough, phlegm-filled:** Sleep with head raised on extra pillow to promote drainage; cough (expectorate) mucus into disposable tissue whenever possible; suck menthol (or other numbing) lozenges; drink herbal teas with honey, other hot water-based beverages to thin mucus.

■ **diarrhea:** Follow clear liquid diet (water or ginger ale, no medication) to rest bowels and replace fluids. If condition is severe, see your doctor. Drink an herbal tea high in tannin content (for a binding effect);

Garlic *Allium sativum*	A perennial herb from lily family with cloved bulb, long flat pointed leaves, pink/white flowers, imported from Europe, now widely grown in U.S. Bulb used in dried form, raw, or to make extracts, oil, powder.	A centuries-old antibacterial, used as remedy for colds, sore throats, coughs, respiratory conditions. Also thought to have expectorant qualities. used in gargles and tea for this purpose. Applied directly to skin for relief of aching joints. High in vitamins A, B₁, B₂, C. Cotton ball soaked in garlic oil and placed in ear is old remedy for ear infections.
Ginger *Zingiber officinale*	A 2- to 4-foot tall exotic tropical plant with cane stalk, swordlike leaves, aromatic flower, grown in tropical climes, notably Jamaica. Root or rhizome—called gingerroot—used in oils, extracts, dried form, powders.	A classic remedy for colds, flu, coughs, invigorating tea made from fresh root helps eliminate mucus, reduce nausea. Hot ginger tea helps get rid of chills; compresses on head relieve sinus, on chest relieve congestion from colds, flu, bronchitis and other pulmonary complaints. Ginger-soaked cotton ball useful for earache relief. Applied to skin it increases blood circulation, thus helps relieve aches, pains of flu.
Peppermint *Mentha piperita*	A perennial herb from mint family with toothy, oblong stalked leaves, lilac/pink long-blooming flowers, native to Europe but now prolific in North America. First cousin of spearmint. Leaves fresh and dried, used in extracts, oil.	Remedy for coughs, pulmonary complaints, treatment of cold... perspiration to break fevers; stimulates circulation ... good gargle for sore throats or rub for achi... peppermint tea at first sign of co... tea soothes dry cough ... expectorant ... OTC ...

can te...
during...
carry...
Chew...

a...
t...

include bananas and rice in your diet (for their binding effect) when you resume solid foods; try herbal solutions containing garlic, goldenseal, slippery elm.

■ **earache:** See your doctor for what is possibly a bacterial infection associated with your cold or flu. In the meantime, sit upright so the ear can drain; yawn to flex muscle that opens eustachian tubes connecting ear to back of throat; do *not* use hot water bottle: Blood vessels swell with heat (try ice pack instead to open ear cavity); keep body moist, room humid; try steamy shower; use anti-inflammatory analgesic to decrease secretion, shrink mucous membranes, and reduce pain; try herbals that include echinacea.

■ **eye irritation:** Tear mechanism that usually soothes, cleans, and lubricates eye may be irritated or dry as a result of your cold or flu. Lubricate with artificial tears. Colds often cause conjunctivitis, an inflammation of the conjunctiva, or thin membrane covering the inner eyelid, and white of the eye that is filled with many blood vessels that dilate and fill with blood. To soothe and shrink blood vessels, flush with Murine or Visine and take a decongestant. Try herbals that contain barberry or goldenseal (sometimes mixed with a dilution of fennel and boric acid in an eyewash).

■ **fatigue:** Rest or sleep until you don't feel tired. If you don't feel like sleeping or staying in bed, get up and move around, but tone down your normal pace; drink ginseng herbal tea for energy.

■ **fever:** Let a fever of 101° or below run its course without medication. If discomfort is extreme and you need to medicate, take an analgesic every three to four hours, especially in the afternoon and evening, which will prevent fever from fluctuating up and down; drink fluids; rest or stay in bed; try fever-lowering herbals and foods.

■ **glands, swollen** (actually, swollen lymph nodes and salivary glands in neck area): A frequent sore throat or ear infection accompaniment, swollen glands if sore and tender, may indicate bacterial infection that requires an antibiotic, so call your doctor; otherwise, no treatment is required. Swollen lymph nodes often take longer than other cold or flu symptoms to subside, but if they don't reduce in size after two weeks following a cold or flu, see your doctor.

■ **headache:** Analgesics every four hours, as needed and advised by your doctor. For sinus headache relief: Apply cold packs to forehead and just below eyes, above teeth. If hot packs feel better, use heat. Try acupressure; steamy shower; salt-water nasal syringe treatment; for sinus headaches, try herbals that include ephedra, caffeine, or eucalyptus (don't take in combination with a decongestant).

■ **hoarseness (laryngitis):** Rest your vocal cords; breathe moist air from a humidifier, vaporizer, or shower; drink plenty of fluids; don't smoke; suck anesthetizing lozenges; drink herbal tea with honey; gargle. This condition may stay longer than the active part of your cold, but if it persists more than two weeks, see your doctor.

■ **nasal congestion:** Blow your nose gently, often; use saline syringe or spray to flush nasal area; take a decongestant, preferably in spray form or nose drops, if your discomfort dictates that you medicate; do not use topical spray or inhalant for more than three days; dab mentholated salve under nostril; keep house and bedroom humidified; drink plenty of fluids (preferably hot). Try herbals (in hot tea form, if possible) that include: slippery elm, eucalyptus or menthol, ephedra, or caffeine.

■ **nausea:** Try a bismuth-based medication (like Pepto-Bismol), ginger- or peppermint-based herbals; don't force foods, especially fats; sip clear liquids slowly, in small quantities that include simple salts and sugars (to restore electrolytes); avoid acidic citrus juices; let carbonated beverages go "flat" first to avoid further distention of your stomach; try an herbal tea.

■ **sinusitis:** If it appears this is a bacterial sinus infection, see your doctor for an antibiotic course of treatment. Otherwise, take analgesics to reduce pain, inflammation; use a decongestant; drink an 8-ounce glass of water or "thin" fruit juice (as opposed to a mucilaginous juice, which coats the throat and can add to drainage congestion) every hour or two; use a bulb syringe with salt water rinse; apply cold or hot packs to affected sinus areas; keep house moist; try steamy showers; use acupressure; try menthol- or eucalyptus-containing herbals and hot herbal tea decoctions.

■ **throat, sore:** Be sure you do not have a strep throat. Drink warm or hot fluids, including herbal tea with honey, to soothe; suck on menthol, eucalyptus, benzocaine or phenol lozenges to numb and moisten; keep room moist; gargle with salt water rinse to reduce inflammation and promote healing; try herbal recipes containing mint or thyme. As a last resort for pain, take an analgesic.

■ **weakness:** Rest; monitor your food intake to include proteins whenever you go back to solid foods (if you have been on a liquid diet); take vitamin supplements.

■ **wheezing:** If you have asthma or another chronic lung condition, see your doctor immediately. Don't smoke and avoid being around tobacco smoke; drink plenty of fluids; introduce moisture to your surroundings using a vaporizer or humidifier; take a steamy shower; suck on lozenges.

4 On the Horizon

Will the dawn of the 21st century bring a cold or flu cure? Research efforts were greatly diminished in 1972 when federal funding for finding a cold vaccine was dropped. Since then, viral researchers and epidemiologists along with various major pharmaceutical companies have diligently pursued several avenues of exploration, funded by private grants. While a number of the experiments in progress show promise (and some drugs are now in multiyear trials), the search for a cold or flu cure is overshadowed by these inhibiting factors:

■ **Money is tight.** Major funding for cold research doesn't exist. And, even though flu and colds are the nation's costliest illnesses in terms of time lost and money invested in cold relief, they are still considered "minor illnesses." Consumers are not willing to spend big dollars on a cold cure (estimates for some experimental antiviral drugs run as high as $250 per cold).

■ **Drug-staying power is limited.** Promising cold drugs under development—nasal sprays, for instance—fall victim to the fact that those with colds or flu fully blow their noses an average of every 15 minutes during the waking day—and, to date, no substance that kills off nasal symptoms of a cold or flu can do it that quickly, even with repeated applications.

■ **Side effects inhibit further use of some new drugs** that appear to work well on the cold or flu itself. People are much less tolerant of a drug's side effects if it's used to treat a minor illness.

■ **Transition from test tube to real life has seen some failures.** Numbers of experiments on flu and cold symptom reduction have recorded great success in vitro—in the test tube—but they have failed to make the transition to clinical human trials.

All of the negatives notwithstanding, the most promising cold and flu research does continue. For more information on the four main areas of cold and flu research, see the Appendix.

when inhaled, and joint pain when injected. Hot paprika made from hot chili peppers is high in natural aspirin.

■ **coffee:** Contains psychoactive drug caffeine, a remedy for asthma and chest congestion (dilates bronchial passages); in moderation, gives sedative effect.

■ **cranberry:** Strong antiviral, antibiotic properties; unusual abilities to prevent infectious bacteria from sticking to cells lining bladder and urinary tract.

■ **licorice:** Kills bacteria, fights diarrhea, but can raise blood pressure.

■ **mushrooms (Asian, including shitake):** Antiviral flu treatment. Contain broad-spectrum antiviral phytochemical compounds that aid immune function.

■ **mustard (including horseradish):** Decongestant/expectorant, breaks up mucus in air passages. Remedy for congestion caused by colds, sinus problems.

■ **onion (including shallots, yellow, red, not white):** Powerful anti-inflammatory, antiviral, antioxidant with strong phytochemical sedative; fights asthma, chronic bronchitis, infections.

■ **pineapple:** Antiviral among other healing attributes; has enzyme that suppresses inflammation.

■ **plum:** Antiviral, laxative.

■ **raspberry:** Antiviral, high in natural aspirin.

■ **rice:** Antidiarrheal.

■ **seaweed (kelp):** Antiviral that boosts immune functioning; high in iodine, so some people may have reactions to it.

■ **soybean:** Active antiviral agent.

■ **strawberry:** Antiviral.

■ **tea (including black, oolong, and green, but not herbals):** Ingredient catechin makes it antibiotic, antidiarrheal, antiviral; ingredient caffeine makes it diuretic, analgesic, and a mild sedative.

■ **turmeric:** Anti-inflammatory agent on par with cortisone; studies show it reduces inflammation in animals, and arthritis symptoms in humans; boosts stomach defenses against acid.

■ **Garlic:** Take two to three capsules a day of this natural immune system enhancer.

■ **B-complex vitamins:** Increase in a multivitamin over your normal daily intake, taking 50-100 mg., three times a day.

Check with your practitioner about any nutritional supplements you plan to take.

72 Eat these everyday infection-fighting foods.

You've heard that eating foods containing essential vitamins does more for you than popping a vitamin supplement. New research underscores the idea that whole foods, especially fruits and vegetables, contain thousands of natural disease-fighting compounds called phytochemicals that boost the efficacy of the food's vitamin contents. In *Food: Your Miracle Medicine*, Carper reviews everyday foods that help you get well when you have a cold or the flu. In its April 25, 1994, issue, *Newsweek* published an in-depth look at the world of phytochemical research, citing common foods that contain miracle compounds that help you get rid of viruses. Here are highlights of foods associated with colds and flu:

■ **bananas and plantains:** Soothe upset stomach, strengthen stomach lining against acid; antibiotic.

■ **bell peppers:** Help immune system fight colds, asthma, bronchitis, respiratory infections; high in vitamin C.

■ **blueberry:** Blocks the attachment of bacteria-causing chemicals; curbs diarrhea; antiviral activity; high in natural aspirin.

■ **cabbage and cauliflower:** Cruciferous vegetables with antiviral powers; well-known antioxidants, abundant in numerous strong phytochemical compounds.

■ **carrot:** Immune-boosting, infection-fighting antioxidant containing beta carotene.

■ **chili peppers:** Antibacterials, antioxidants; open sinuses, air passages, break up mucus in lungs; expectorants and decongestants; prevent bronchitis; phytochemical properties from capsaicin, the compound that makes peppers hot. Painkillers, alleviate headaches

another, carried out in 1987 by cold researcher Jack M. Gwaltney Jr.,
M.D., at the University of Virginia Medical Center, showed that zinc
lozenges had no pronounced beneficial effects on shortening the
cold's duration.

Zinc does have a significant effect on strengthening the immune
system, however. A new study by Ananda S. Prasad, M.D., of Wayne
State University School of Medicine, reported in the March 23, 1994,
Star-Ledger, focused on 118 healthy 50-to-80-year-olds. The 30 percent
who had zinc deficiencies also had lower immunity.

A word of caution: Prolonged zinc overdosing can lead to
cholesterol, heart, and thyroid problems. Opinion on how much zinc
is too much is divided, so we suggest that, if you're thinking about
taking zinc lozenges, you seek your doctor's recommendations.

71 Adjust your vitamins when you have a cold or flu.

Studies show that increasing vitamin and mineral supplements when you have a cold or flu can have some
positive results. The added vitamin and mineral punch may help
shorten duration and severity of your illness. There are many schools
of thought concerning which in particular to augment.

Here's a vitamin diet, adjusted for an adult with a cold or flu,
recommended by James F. Balch, M.D., in Prescription for Nutritional
Healing*. He advises reducing the normal food diet and increasing fluid
intake. Then, he says, take the following daily doses of supplements:

■ **Vitamin A:** 15,000 I.U. plus 15,000 I.U. of beta carotene (to
help heal inflamed mucous membranes and strengthen the immune system);

■ **Vitamin C:** 5,000-10,000 mg., in divided doses (to destroy
cold viruses);

■ **Zinc gluconate lozenges:** Dissolve one under the tongue every
three hours during the first three days of a cold or flu, then drop to one
every four hours for a week.

---

*Garden City Park, N.Y.: Avery, 1990.

Whole Foods, studies show that if you take it in combination with bio-flavonoids (phytochemicals found just under the rind in citrus fruits, among other places), vitamin C gets a boost that can reduce the duration of a cold or the flu by as much as 50 percent.

Augmenting vitamin C when you have a cold or flu gains support from leading cold researcher Elliott Dick, M.D., of the University of Wisconsin, whose study in the 1980s found that cold sufferers taking 500 mg. of vitamin C four times a day had only half as many symptoms as those not taking vitamin C at all. (In three separate 1991 trials, Dick found that vitamin C did not prevent infection but "markedly, consistently, and significantly reduced signs and symptoms of rhinovirus colds," he told *American Health* in 1993.)

Since vitamin C is an acid, multiple grams of it may not appeal to you or sit well with your stomach. (Effects of overdosing vary from individual to individual and include diarrhea, nausea, and/or stomach pains.) But it's important to take enough to make a difference: Researchers suggest that several clinical studies on the effects of vitamin C were inconclusive because volunteers took too few milligrams (under 250 mg./day) to count.

70 Try taking zinc gluconate lozenges.

Taking the mineral zinc almost immediately stimulates antibody and T-cell production and helps fuel circulation of the white blood cells that rid the body of cold and flu viruses. In 1984 University of Texas researchers conducted clinical studies in which people with common colds dissolved a 23-mg. zinc lozenge or a matched placebo in the mouth every two wakeful hours. After seven days, 86 percent of the zinc-taking subjects were free of cold symptoms, compared to only 46 percent of the placebo-treated subjects. They concluded that zinc lozenges shortened the average duration of common colds by about a week.*

Not all zinc lozenge experiments have had the same good results, however. One conducted at the University of Pennsylvania and

---

*Feltman, John, ed. *Prevention's How-To Dictionary of Healing Remedies and Techniques.* Emmaus, Pa.: Rodale, 1992.

■ APPENDIX
Promising Cold and
Flu Research

As mentioned in Chapter 4, there are four principal areas of cold and flu research. They are as follows:

1 ■ Developing molecular alterations that keep cold and flu viruses from attaching to human cells or that immobilize the virus itself.

Recent breakthrough x-ray **crystallography imaging** led by Purdue University's Michael G. Rossmann, M.D., showed scientists a rhinovirus in three dimensions for the first time. This opened doors to understanding the complex structure of the most prominent cold virus and how it attaches to host human cells.

Capsid binders are drugs under development that would prevent rhinovirus from attacking host cells. Molecules that block binding sites on human nose and throat cells would make it impossible for a rhinovirus to enter and corrupt a human cell. Rossmann has been working to find a drug that stiffens the viral cell coating so that it can't commandeer human cells. These **uncoating inhibitors** would also change the virus molecule, preventing them from attaching to human cells.

One **receptor-blocker** has been tested by Merck with encouraging results. Those treated with the drug who were then exposed to a rhinovirus developed their cold symptoms several days later than the control group, and their symptoms were less severe. The downside to the trials, according to a January 29, 1990, report in *U.S. News & World Report*, was that the human immune system subsequently destroyed the drug.

Seeking to prevent Type A flu, Milton J. Schlesinger, Ph.D., of Washington University in St. Louis, designed a molecular peptide that alters the flu virus itself—blocking attachment of its Velcro-like spikes to itself—which consequently prevents it from entering the host cell. With mobility restricted, the virus can then be killed by the immune system. The 1991 test-tube results were 95 percent effective. Schlesinger is continuing his work on the **peptide blocker** under partial sponsorship from the National Institutes of Health.

Agouron Pharmaceuticals announced the discovery in January 1994 of the atomic structure of the enzyme *rhinovirus 3C protease*, a principal cause of rhinovirus colds. They are conducting research to develop an antiviral that will **inhibit replication** of the cold-causing enzyme.

Under this approach, **decoy receptor molecules** are introduced in huge quantity into the nose by a drug, then they lure away and incapacitate the invading virus. In 1990 the British journal *Nature* reported on a joint British-American study that successfully developed a synthetic form of the human nasal molecule to which an invading virus attaches. In test tubes the synthetic decoy was able to attract and block the virus. Questions yet to be answered concern whether the decoy also affects nonviral cells and whether the substance will succeed out of the clinical medium. Researchers did not expect trials to begin before 1995.

2 ■ Developing drugs that diminish or eradicate cold or flu symptoms once the virus has entered the body.

Alpha interferon, a synthetic copy of the body's natural virus-fighting, immune-boosting substance, was developed into a **nasal spray** in 1986. *Consumer Reports Health Letter* reported in December 1990 that, in trials, it reduced the spread of all colds by 40 percent and rhinovirus colds by 80 percent. But side effects of interferon—nasal dryness, stuffiness, minor nasal bleeding—occurred in 10 percent of users by the end of the first week and up to 50 percent after two to four weeks. Cost, too, was prohibitive.

In 1992 University of Virginia viral researcher Jack M. Gwaltney Jr., M.D., conducted a controlled study testing an **antiviral compound** using interferon and two anti-inflammatory drugs, ipratropium and naproxen. The drug reduced contagion and lightened cold symptoms of those treated. It also prevented colds from developing in many and reduced colds' severity in others. But study continues: The compound is currently too expensive to bring to market.

Concurrent studies in which Gwaltney has also participated center on the discovery of a chemical released from nasal cells called bradykinins, which are thought to cause cold symptoms to occur and stimulate pain receptor activity. Experiments have focused on finding a **bradykinin blocker**—a substance to either block its release or to stop it from acting. Doctors from Johns Hopkins University have been working with Gwaltney on an interferon nasal spray (NPC 567) containing a bradykinin antagonist that blocks cold symptoms. According to the November 1993 *American Health*, trials succeeded in reducing severe cold symptoms and were free of side effects. FDA approval is anticipated within two to three years.

3 ■ Expanding or redirecting use of currently approved medications for control and/or prevention of colds and flu.

NIH reports that **rimantadine**, a new drug coming to the U.S. market and related to amantadine (currently used to lessen the effects of Type A flu and viral pneumonia), is effective in preventing and treating Type A flu reportedly with fewer side effects. Researchers are looking into the efficacy (and costs) of high-risk patients taking the medication daily during flu season, as a preventative.

George Washington University researchers promote an **aspirin** a day for increasing natural, virus-fighting immune substances interferon and interleukin-2, which help fight cold and flu symptoms.

Ribavarin is a new drug that fights respiratory infections by disrupting the viral RNA needed to relay commands to the viral cells. It is helpful, according to early reports, in moderating some colds, but may not be as effective against other classes of cold or flu virus.

4 ■ Developing methods to keep viruses from spreading.

Virologist Elliott Dick, M.D., of the University of Wisconsin, a leading proponent of the airborne theory of cold contagion, developed a facial tissue several years ago permeated with a virus-killing chemical. Clinical trial results were convincing: the **virucidal tissues** dramatically decreased the spread of colds in the trial group. Kimberly-Clark manufacturers joined with him to produce the tissues commercially, but their cost—three times more than standard tissues—made them a disaster in the marketplace.

Now, a 12-year study comes to the attention of flu researchers that some recombined (mutated) virulent flu virus strains carry avianlike genes —viruses from birds. People can't catch flu from birds, but pigs can (invariably, say researchers, where the avian and swine viruses mix and mutate), and people can catch flu viruses from pigs ("swine flu"). New research detailed in the June 1993 Discover suggests that virologists may start looking into the development and administration of a **flu vaccine for pigs.**

Samples of other research underway: The April 13, 1994, Journal of the American Medical Association reports on drug-free experiments administering **heated humidified air** to nasal passages of those with colds to see if higher temperatures can prevent replication of heat-sensitive rhinoviruses. Early clinical trials showed dramatic, positive results but various problems — including inability to conduct unbiased placebo studies — prevail. And one biotechnical company, Shaman Pharmaceuticals, is clinically testing SP-303, an agent derived from **a weedlike tropical plant** from the Amazon, which they told Trends in Health Business is a potent antiviral compound.

■ GLOSSARY/ INDEX

Acupressure: A system of therapy that addresses health problems using finger- and thumb tips to apply pressure and thus stimulate pain or nerve points (meridians) found on the body. (See tips 48, 75, and 77.)

Acupuncture: A system of therapy in which very thin needle points are inserted temporarily under the skin to help relieve pain and restore good health. (See tip 48.)

Aerobic exercise: Exercise designed to increase cardiovascular fitness and endurance in which the body meets the increasing oxygen demand of muscles created by increasing the body's level of activity. (See tips 42, 47, and 68.)

Allergy: Hypersensitivity or overreaction to substances such as pollen, dust, food, or drugs. (See tips 10, 18, 53, 57, and 73.)

Allicin: The natural active antibacterial ingredient of garlic formed when a garlic clove is crushed and alliin—the parent substance—combines with the enzyme allinase. An unstable substance, allicin is partially inactivated when exposed to heat. (See tip 24.)

Amantadine: Short for amantadine hydrochloride, a drug that can prevent one from contracting Type A flu or eradicate Type A flu and certain kinds of pneumonia, if taken early in the course of the illness; associated with strong side effects. (See tip 61.)

Amino acids: Compounds that form the chief constituents of protein. Twenty amino acids are necessary for the body to make protein, a process called protein synthesis. (See tips 24, 25, 29, and 67.)

Analgesic: A drug that relieves pain. (See tips 50, 53, 54, 72, and 77.)

Antibody: A protein manufactured in the body by lymphocytes that fights or neutralizes foreign substances (antigens) in the body. Antibodies attack and try to destroy or incapacitate invading cold and flu viruses. (See tips 28, 29, 49, 57, 68, and 70.)

Antioxidants: Molecules that help limit potentially harmful oxidizing reactions by neutralizing free radicals, the molecular fragments that roam the body, damaging other molecules. Nutrients that act as antioxidants include vitamins C and E, beta carotene, and selenium. (See tips 26, 27, 29, 30, 32, and 72.)

Antipyretic: A drug that reduces fever. (See tips 50 and 53.)

Antitussive: A cough suppressant. (See tips 50, 54, 57, 58, 68, and 77.)

Astringent gargle: A liquid mixture for swilling in the throat that is intended to reduce irritation of a sore throat by constricting (contracting) blood vessels and tissues. (See tip 67.)

Bacteria: Microorganisms that do not cause colds or flu but can cause secondary problems. (See tips 7, 10, 58, 62, 63, 66, 67, 72, and 77.)

Benzocaine: An anesthetic drug derived or synthesized from the benzoin tree that numbs pain and reduces itching. Used externally, it is a major ingredient of many over-the-counter skin irritation and arthritis remedies. (See tips 59 and 77.)

Biotin: A B-complex vitamin, important in the metabolism of protein, carbohydrates, and fat. (See tip 29.)

Bismuth subsalicylate: The drug, derived from salts of the metal bismuth and salicylic acid, found in many over-the-counter drugs; used for settling the stomach and as a remedy for other intestinal inflammations. The drug works by coating irritated areas, which permits healing to take place. (See tip 77.)

Camphor rub: A skin balm made from camphor, a natural ingredient from the camphor tree that is a crystal-like substance with a strong odor and taste. It serves as a mild irritant and helps "open" clogged nasal or upper respiratory passages. (See tip 67.)

Complication: A secondary infection, usually bacterial in nature, that follows a cold or case of flu and that often needs treatment with an antibiotic drug before it can be eradicated from the body. (See tips 18, 20, 31, 32, 60, 62, 63, 67, and 74.)

Crucifers: The vegetables of the cabbage family that include broccoli, cauliflower, brussels sprouts, and kale. They are high in fiber and considered among the most potent phytochemicals in prevention of colon cancers as well as colds and flu. (See tip 72.)

Decongestant: A drug used to reduce congestion or swelling, especially of the nasal passages. (See tips 50, 54, 55, 57, 67, 72, 76, and 77.)

Disinfectant: An antiseptic containing an antibacterial ingredient, which destroys bacteria. (See tips 1, 5, and 9.)

Folic acid: A B vitamin, essential in DNA synthesis, and cell reproduction and growth. (See tip 29.)

Food Guide Pyramid: The pyramid-shaped visual presentation introduced by the U.S. Department of Agriculture to educate people on the currently recognized food groups and how many portions of each should be consumed on a daily basis in order to maintain good health. (See tips 19 and 20.)

Genetic nutrition: An approach to diet and nutrition cited in a 1993 book of the same name in which one designs his or her diet based on inherited (genetic) and environmental factors peculiar to him- or herself in order to enjoy optimal good health. (See tip 21.)

Ginger: A herbaceous flowering tropical plant whose pungent root has been used for centuries for culinary and medical purposes. Ginger is thought to calm the stomach as well as promote sweating and perspiration; thought to be useful in shortening colds. (See tips 25 and 77.)

Ginseng: The active ingredient of a flowering herbaceous plant of the same name whose root has been used for two centuries in herbal mixtures, including teas, that are thought to give energy boosts and cure many ills. (See tips 25 and 77.)

Immune response: A defensive reaction of the body to invading microorganisms, cancer cells, transplanted tissue, and other substances that are recognized as "foreign." When this happens, a variety of body chemicals are activated in the effort to neutralize or destroy the invading particles. (See tips 18, 26, 29, 34, 35, 38, 40, 57, 70, 71, 72, and 74.)

Interleukins: A group of natural proteins found in the body which launch the immune response by catalyzing such actions as the production of B- and fighter T-cells, inflammation and fever, T-cell division, and various cellular growth. (See tips 38 and 40.)

I.U.: International Unit, a unit of measure often applied to vitamins, which implies a biological result. For instance, the minimum dietary requirement of vitamin A is 8,000 I.U. (See tips 29 and 71.)

Kelp: A form of brown seaweed that is rich in vitamins, minerals, and trace elements that contains demulcent—or soothing—qualities often used for relief of nasal passage irritation during colds or the flu. (See tips 25 and 72.)

Lysozyme: An enzyme that destroys microbes and helps break down mucus. (See tip 29.)

Massage: Application of hand manipulation on the body to create relaxation, relieve tension, alleviate aches and pains, and stimulate the body's systems. Different massage forms include shiatsu, acupressure, Swedish, rolfing, and reflexology. (See tips 67 and 77.)

Meditation: Achieving inward concentration that allows a person to clear the mind of thoughts and focus on his or her senses; a form of learned relaxation that stimulates endorphin release. (See tip 49.)

Menthol: An anesthetic derived and/or synthesized from peppermint that numbs pain and reduces itching and other surface irritation of skin and throat. Used in many over-the-counter cough and cold relief drugs. (See tips 59, 67, 68, and 77.)

Meridians: Pathways throughout the body, through which life's energy is thought to flow and which connect the various acupressure/acupuncture points. (See tip 48.)

Mucilaginous: Literally, mucuslike or gluelike and slimy; used in this case to refer to natural ingredients from botanicals whose viscous properties soothe inflammation. (See tips 58, 67, and 77.)

Mucous membrane: A thin sheet of tissue cells that line various parts of the body, including the openings of the passageways of the upper respiratory system; a membrane that releases mucus— a sticky, slippery material consisting of mucin (a carbohydrate), white blood cells, water, and tissue debris. A cold or flu involves inflammation of these linings. (See tips 10, 12, 13, 14, 31, 57, 59, 67, 71, 74, and 77.)

Multi-ingredient cold remedies: Cold relief products, generally sold over-the-counter, that have more than one ingredient, each aimed at eliminating or relieving a different cold or flu symptom. (See tip 54.)

Nasal inhalant: Any substance–drug or natural–intended to be taken into the body by inhaling it through the nose. Over-the-counter nasal inhalants include nasal sprays and nose drops. (See tips 12, 55, 56, 66, 76, and 77.)

Natural food supplements: Products composed of, derived from or by-products of foods that are believed to provide a variety of health benefits. These may help healing, assist a bodily function such as digestion, or provide a combination of nutrients (such as vitamins) and active ingredients. (See tips 24, 27, 28, 29, 30, 71, 72, 73, and 77.)

Neutrophil: An immune system chemical that rushes to the site of an infection, thus helping cause inflammation symptomatic of infections. (See tips 29 and 67.)

Niacin: Also known as vitamin B_3, a B-complex family member that aids in release of energy from foods and helps maintain healthy skin. (See tip 29.)

Nonproductive cough: A dry, hacking cough that produces no phlegm and that thus does not contribute to ending a cold's or flu's symptoms. This kind of cough can be medicated without harming the cold's progress. (See tips 58, 68, and 77.)

OTC: Abbreviation for over-the-counter, referring to drugs dispensed without a doctor's prescription, widely available in drugstores and grocery stores. (See tips 51, 52, 53, and 56.)

Pantothenic acid: Also known as vitamin B_5, a B-complex vitamin that plays a number of essential metabolic roles. (See tip 29.)

Phenol and sodium phenolate compounds: Anesthetic, or numbing, active ingredients contained in many over-the-counter sore throat remedies. (See tips 59 and 77.)

Phytochemical compounds: A newly discovered class of natural compounds found in various fruits and vegetables that are thought to give the accompanying vitamins a super boost. Phytochemicals are being studied for their possible roles in preventing illnesses – from colds to cancers. (See tips 22, 24, 30, 69, and 72.)

Psychoactive drug: A drug that has an effect on the mind. (See tip 72.)

Pyridoxine: A vitamin, also known as vitamin B_6, required for the proper functioning of more than 60 enzymes in the body, including those necessary for the body's metabolism of proteins, fats, and carbohydrates. (See tip 29.)

Reishi (shitake) mushrooms: A natural ingredient, used in cooking (dry or powdered forms); used to build resistance to viral infection. They contain a virus that stimulates interferon production. (See tips 25 and 72.)

Relative humidity: Ratio of actual water vapor in the air at a specific temperature to the maximum capacity of the air at that temperature. (See tip 10.)

Royal jelly: A honey and pollen derivative, especially high in the B vitamins, containing vitamins A, C, D, E, and an array of minerals and amino acids. Boosts the immune system response. (See tip 25.)

Saline nasal spray: A nonmedical nasal spray made of salt and water; used to moisturize nasal cavity and flush allergens and germs from nose. (See tips 12, 66, and 77.)

Self-inoculation: Refers to infecting oneself (for instance, with a cold) by touching a cold-contaminated person or object, then touching one's own nose, eyes, or mouth, thereby transmitting the germ to oneself. (See tip 1.)

Single-ingredient cough or cold remedy: A drug–either prescription or over-the-counter–that attacks only one symptom or attempts to achieve one result. For instance, a cough suppressant is a single-ingredient cough remedy that is intended to stop or suppress coughing. (See tips 54 and 68.)

Strep throat: An infection of the throat and tonsils caused by a bacterium. The infection is marked by sore throat, fever, chills, swollen lymph nodes in the neck, and, sometimes, nausea and vomiting. (See tips 60, 62, and 77.)

Sulforaphane: A tumor-blocking substance known as a phytochemical found in broccoli, cauliflower, brussels sprouts, and kale. (See tip 22.)

Systemic: Affecting the entire body. For instance, an oral decongestant is systemic, but a nasal spray is localized. (See tip 55.)

T-cell production: The activity prompted by interleukins as a major part of the immune response, in which these cells are reproduced for the purpose of killing or neutralizing the invading germs. (See tip 70.)

Tannin: A natural ingredient of many teas; a chemical used to stop bleeding and control diarrhea as well as to stop the tickle in a sore throat. (See tips 67 and 77.)

Thiamin: Also called vitamin B_1, a nutrient essential for energy metabolism and for nearly every cellular reaction taking place in the body–for normal development, growth, reproduction, maximum physical fitness, and good health. (See tip 29.)

Timed-release medicines: Any drug that is intended to break down and disperse through the body over an extended period of time, rather than all at once. They are intended to have sustained effects. (See tip 54.)

Upper respiratory infection (URI): The term physicians use for a cold whose symptoms are generally limited to the head. (See tips 67 and 72.)

Vaporizer: A machine that disperses hot or cold water vapors into the air for the purpose of keeping moisture in a room. (See tips 67 and 77.)

Viruses: Submicroscopic organisms that cause disease, including colds and flu. A virus is a parasite that cannot reproduce on its own: It invades a host cell and commandeers the host's genetic material as its own by breaking down the host cell's molecular structure and merging with it. In its reproductive process, a virus destroys the host cell. (See tips 1, 2, 3, 4, 6, 7, 8, 10, 14, 15, 16, 17, 18, 21, 22, 24, 27, 28, 29, 32, 35, 36, 38, 43, 47, 50, 58, 62, 66, 68, 69, 70, 71, 72, and 74.)

Vitamin C: Also known as ascorbate or ascorbic acid, a water-soluble vitamin with strong antioxidant properties. Helps to protect against cancer and heart disease, boosts immune function, speeds wound healing, and provides numerous other benefits. (See tips 22, 25, 26, 27, 29, 30, 32, 69, 71, and 72.)

Zinc gluconate lozenges: Lozenges impregnated with a compound containing the mineral zinc, thought by some to have cold-relieving properties. (See tips 70 and 71.)